# Plant Based Diet Guide for Beginners

*A step by step plant-based diet guide for beginners: the plant-based diet made easy, with vegan and vegetarian tips. 21 days meal plan included*

# Table of Contents

**Chapter 5.    Dinner recipes .................................................................189**

# Introduction

A plant-based keto Diet Plan is very limiting.

The plant-based keto diet regimen is doable, yet it may difficult to manage depending on how rigorous your decision to follow through is.

Attempting to be vegan while following a keto diet may present some real obstacles, consisting of unsustainable weight loss, eating too little calories, and nutrient deficiencies.

Protein is vital for your wellness, and the restrictions of healthy protein sources on a plant-based keto diet might leave you at risk for a shortage.

If you wish to try this diet, ensure you're on top of your healthy protein intake, followed by a lot of healthy fats.

It might supply some wellness advantages as well, such as rapid fat burning and a decrease in body fat. Similar to a vegan diet plan, a vegan keto diet regimen might provide some benefits to the wellness of the heart.

Nevertheless, it is a highly restrictive diet plan that is not ideal for every person. The diet plan carries certain risks, consisting of the risk of creating dietary shortages.

Some people may additionally experience damaging consequences, such as headaches and tiredness, at the beginning.

It is crucial to plan a vegan keto diet plan meticulously and to take dietary supplements to prevent shortages. Due to the restrictive nature of this diet regimen, individuals that want to try it out, ought to talk to a physician.

The reality is that moms and dads were right: We all require to eat our veggies. Meat and dairy products, on the other hand, can be disposed of. The evidence remains in the present state of wellness in wealthy countries where meat and dairy preponderate, we find an epidemic of diabetes, excessive weight, heart problems, and cancer.

Look at it this way: How many plant-based eaters do you know of that have died of nutrient deficiencies? What is the number of meat-eaters that you know of who have died as a result of diet-related concerns? What is the bigger problem?

# Chapter 1. Benefits of the plant based diet

Benefits of a Plant-based Diet. Choose the One for You.

A plant-based diet has significant benefits of improving health and being eco-friendlier. Some of the benefits are as follows:

Weight Loss and Overall Improved Health

Obesity is one of the significant health issues faced by the majority of people these days, ranging from children to old. Proper diet changes can lead to radical weight loss, which would be promising and long-lasting. Various studies report that effective weight loss can be achieved with the help of plant-based diet plans.

The plant-based diet plan is ideal for weight loss, as it is rich in proteins and fiber, limits processed foods, and forbids refined grains, soda, candy, fast food, and added sugars. According to a few research reports, plant-based diet followers lose weight more quickly as compared to non-plant-based diet followers. Weight loss from a plant-based diet plan is quite long-lasting with improved health.

Beneficial in Various Health Issues

In addition to weight loss, a plant-based diet helps to reduce the menaces of numerous chronic health conditions.

## Cardiac Conditions

The foremost benefit of a plant-based diet plan is that it keeps the cardiac health sound, depending upon the quality and types of the food in your diet plan. Research studies report that the risk of cardiac diseases was lower in those people who follow a plant-based diet that was rich in veggies, whole grains, nuts, fruits, and legumes, as compared to followers of other diets. Plant-based diet plans, including refined grains, sugary drinks, and fruit juices, are very unhealthy and contribute to severe cardiac complications. So, it is essential to follow a healthy plant-based diet plan.

## Cancer

Research studies report that a plant-based diet plan can avoid various forms of cancer. The risks of gastrointestinal and colorectal cancers are reported to be significantly reduced amongst plant-based diet followers.

## Cognitive Decline

According to some studies, Alzheimer's disease and cognitive decline can be prevented in adults with the help of diet plans high in veggie and fruit content due to a large number of antioxidants and other compounds. Consumption of more fruits and vegetables leads to a 20 percent lower risk of having dementia or cognitive impairment.

## Diabetes

In order to reduce the risk of contracting diabetes, one should consider following a plant-based diet plan. Followers of the plant-based diet plan mitigate the risk of having diabetes by 34 percent when compared to followers of other diets. Fifty percent reduction of type 2 diabetes was observed amongst the followers of Lacto-Ovo vegetarian and vegan diet plans. Blood sugar level control is highly improved in the diabetic followers of plant-based diet plans.

Eco-friendlier Diet

In addition to benefits in health, a plant-based diet plan has proved to be advantageous for the ecosystem, as they have little effect on the environment as compared to other diet plan followers. A plant-based diet helps in the minimization of global warming, as it results in a 50-70 percent reduction in greenhouse gas emissions, land usage, and lower water usage. A plant-based diet also helps in boosting the economy due to lower dependency on unsustainable practices like factory farming and reduction in animal-based food.

# Chapter 2. How to approach the plant-based diet

There is a never-ending debate about the best diet suitable for the human body. Nonetheless, the overall health and wellness communities have come to the conclusion that diets which lay much emphasis on the fresh, whole ingredients, while minimizing processed foods have far many superior qualities needed by humans for overall wellness.

The whole-foods, plant-based diet addresses all of this by focusing solely on minimally processed foods, with specifics to plants, which is successful when it comes to weight control and improving our health.

Therefore, we shall look at ways in which we delve much deeper into the world of plant-based whole diets, including all the potential benefits that come with it, what to eat, including a sample meal plan in the end.

What Is a Whole-Foods, Plant-Based Diet?

There is no clear demarcation as to what constitutes a whole-food, otherwise known as a plant-based diet : WFPB diet). This diet is not necessarily set; instead, it is more of a lifestyle where people strive to live healthily.

The main reason why it is so is plant-based diets do vary in an exceptional manner depending on the length in which a person includes animal products in their meals. Nevertheless, the fundamental principles associated with whole-foods, plant-based diet have been highlighted below:

- Emphasizes more on the whole while minimizing processed foods.

- Limits or avoids the intake of animal products.

- Focuses more on plants, including vegetables, fruits, whole grains, legumes, seeds, and nuts, which make up the main ingredients of what you eat.

- Exclusion of refined foods, like added sugars, white flour inclusive of processed oils.

- Special attention is paid to the quality of food. Many advocates of the WFPB diet promoting locally sourced, organic food anytime possible.

It is such principles that make this diet to be confused with vegan or vegetarian diets. Even though they are similar in several ways, both are not the same.

Adherents of vegan diets typically abstain from consuming any animal products, which include eggs, meat, poultry, dairy, seafood, and honey. Vegetarians exclude all poultry and meat from their diets. However, a good number of vegetarians eat eggs, seafood, or dairy.

On the other hand, the WFPB diet is more flexible, whereby Its followers strictly adhere to, but animal products can also be consumed.

In some instances, one person following a WFPB diet may indulge in no animal products; another may as well eat it in smaller quantities, including small amounts of eggs, poultry, seafood, meat, or dairy.

In summary, plant-based whole-foods puts more emphasis on plant-based meals while minimizing processed items and animal products.

It Can Help You Improve Your Health & Lose Weight

Obesity has become a crisis in our lives today, with epidemic proportions. It has been reported that close to over 69% of US adults is overweight or obese. Hence, embarking on dietary measures and making lifestyle adjustments can significantly help in facilitating weight loss, capable of having a positive and lasting impact on your health.

Many studies have also shown how plant-based diets are beneficial when it comes to weight loss. Due to its high fiber content, the WFPB diet, except for processed foods, can be a winning combination for shedding those stubborn and excess pounds

It Benefits Several Health Conditions

When you consume whole-foods, plant-based diet, one of the key benefits will be your waistline; it can also lower the risk while reducing the chances of symptoms of some chronic diseases

Heart Disease

This is perhaps one of the most common benefits of this type of diet is that it is very healthy. However, when it comes to such diets, what you eat matters a lot in a big way in terms of quality.

A study done on large groups of people of over 200,000, found out that those who strictly adhered to a healthy plant-based diet rich in vegetables, fruits, whole-grains, legumes, and nuts posed a significantly lower risk of having heart disease than those who did not use plant-based foods.

On the contrary, those who engaged in unhealthy plant-based diets, which included sugary drinks, fruit juices, and refined grains were at significant risks of suffering from heart disease. That is why consuming the right types of food is very important when it comes to the prevention of heart disease. More so, when you are following a plant-based diet, which is why adhering to a WFPB diet is the best choice that you will ever make.

Cancer

Research has also shown that strict adherence to a plant-based diet may also reduce your risk of suffering from certain types of cancer.

A study done in over 69,000 people revealed that vegetarian diets had a significantly lower risk of getting gastrointestinal cancer. This was especially true for those who adhered to a Lacto-Ovo vegetarian diet. These are vegetarians whose foods include eggs and dairy products.

On the other hand, another large study was conducted by more than 77,000 people, and it showed that those people who followed vegetarian diets had a 22% lower risk of suffering from colorectal cancer than non-vegetarians.

Pescatarians, these are vegetarians who eat fish, had the most considerable amounts of protection from colorectal cancer with a 43% reduction risk as compared to non-vegetarians.

Cognitive Decline

Some studies have even shown that diets, which are very rich in vegetables and fruits, may come in handy in slowing or preventing cognitive decline such as Alzheimer's disease, which is most common in older adults.

Additionally, plant-based diets also have a higher total number of plant compounds and antioxidants. These have been shown to help significantly in slowing down the ravaging effects and progression of Alzheimer's disease.

However, some studies have also shown that higher intakes of fruits and vegetables have an active link to a reduction in cognitive decline.

A review done on about nine studies, which included close to over 31,000 respondents concluded that eating more fruits and vegetables led to a 20% reduction in the risk of suffering from cognitive impairment or dementia for that matter.

Diabetes

Another immense benefit that you might get with this kind of diet is its effectiveness in managing and reducing the risk associated with diabetes.

A study involving more than 200,000 respondents also showed that those who observed a healthy plant-based eating schedule posed a 34% lower risk of having diabetes or its complications altogether, more than those who ate unhealthy and non-plant-based meals.

Significantly, another study also showed that plant-based diets, which are vegan and Lacto-Ovo vegetarian was linked to nearly a 50% reduction when it came to the risk of type 2 diabetes when they were compared to non-vegetarian diets. Besides, plant-based diets have also been used to control blood sugar levels in people who have diabetes.

Foods to Eat on Whole-Foods, Plant-Based Diet

Whether it is eggs and bacon for breakfast or steak for dinner, animal products are usually the most preferred diets in most people's meals almost daily. When you want to make a switch to a plant-based diet, then your meals must focus more on plant-based foods.

And if it is a must that you have to eat animal products, then you should do so in smaller quantities, while paying great attention to its quality.

Food products like dairy, eggs, poultry, meat, and seafood should only be used more as a supplement in regards to a plant-based meal, and not as the main focal point.

Whole-Foods, Plant-Based Shopping List For Beginners

• Fruits: Here, we have berries, citrus fruits, pears, peaches, pineapple, and bananas.

• Vegetables: We shall have here kale, spinach, tomatoes, broccoli, cauliflower, carrots, asparagus, and peppers, among others.

• Starchy vegetables: These include potatoes, sweet potatoes, butternut squash, etc.

• Whole grains: We can find here brown rice, rolled oats, farro, quinoa, brown rice pasta, and barley.

• Healthy fats: These include avocados, olive oil, coconut oil, and unsweetened coconut.

• Legumes: This category has some peas, chickpeas, lentils, peanuts, and black beans.

• Seeds, nuts and nut butter: here we find recipes like almonds, cashews, macadamia nuts, pumpkin seeds, sunflower seeds, natural peanut butter, and tahini, etc.

- Unsweetened plant-based milk: We have coconut milk, almond milk, cashew milk, among other delicious ingredients.

- Spices, herbs, and seasonings: Basil, rosemary, turmeric, curry, black pepper, and salt, etc.

- Condiments: Include Salsa, mustard, nutritional yeast, soy sauce, vinegar, lemon juice, etc.

- Plant-based protein: In this section, we have tofu, tempeh, and plant-based protein sources or powders, which have no added sugar or artificial ingredients.

- Beverages: We shall commonly include coffee, tea, sparkling water, etc.

In case you want to supplement your plant-based diet with animal products, then it is for you to choose quality products from grocery stores or, better still, you can buy them directly from local farms.

- Eggs: Pasture-raised when there is a possibility.

- Poultry: Free-range and organic, where possible.

- Beef and pork: Pastured or grass-fed in nature where possible.

- Seafood: These are wildly-caught from sustainable fisheries.

- Dairy: Organic dairy products derived from pasture-raised animals whenever possible.

Foods To Avoid Or Minimize On This Diet

As a proponent of the WFPB diet, your primary focus should be on how to consume the variety of plant-based meals in their most natural form. This means that you omit any contact or indulgence in heavily processed foods. And in case you are going to purchase your groceries; your main aim should be on fresh foods and, while buying foods that have been labeled; you should strictly aim for items, which have the fewest possible ingredients.

Foods to Avoid

• Fast food: Include French fries, cheeseburgers, hot dogs, chicken nuggets, etc.

• Added sugars and sweets: Here, you shall find table sugar, juice, pastries, cookies, candy, sweet tea, and sugary cereals, etc.

• Refined grains: White rice, white pasta, white bread, and bagels.

• Packaged and convenience foods: You cannot miss finding in this category chips, crackers, cereal bars, frozen dinners, etc.

•   Processed vegan-friendly foods: Will include plant-based meats like Tofurkey, faux cheeses, and vegan butter, capable of enticing you.

• Artificial sweeteners: These are equal, Splenda, Sweeten Low, etc.

• Processed animal products: These include bacon, lunch meats, sausage, and beef jerky, among others.

Foods to Minimize

While healthy animal foods can, at times, be included in such kinds of a diet; you should keep at a minimum such products in all plant-based diets. They include:

- Seafood

- Beef

- Pork

- Mutton

- Game meats

- Poultry products

- Eggs

- Dairy products

Sample Meal Plan for A Week

It does not have to be a tedious affair when transitioning to a whole-food, plant-based diet.

The menu one-week sample menu below can help give you a head start and a rough idea to help you come up with your successful recipe for your favorite ingredients. However, this sample menu is inclusive of a small number of animal products. However, the extent to which you include these foods in your diet will greatly depend upon you.

Monday

• Breakfast: Your breakfast will include a simple recipe of oatmeal made of coconut milk topped with berries, coconut, and walnuts.

• Lunch: On a Monday, lunch will have a salad topped up with fresh vegetables, chickpeas, avocado, pumpkin seeds, and some goat cheese.

• Dinner: Here, you can make do with butternut squash curry.

Tuesday

• Breakfast: Your second day of the week has a full-fat plain yogurt, which can be topped up with sliced strawberries, unsweetened coconut, and or pumpkin seeds.

• Lunch: A sumptuous meatless chili.

• Dinner: A delicious, simple meal of sweet potato and black bean tacos.

Wednesday

• Breakfast: On the third day, you can have a smoothie made of unsweetened coconut milk, berries, peanut butter inclusive of unsweetened plant-based protein powder.

• Lunch: Hummus and veggie wrap.

• Dinner: A simple meal of zucchini noodles tossed in pesto with delicious chicken meatballs.

Thursday

- Breakfast: On the fourth day, you can savor oatmeal with slices of avocado, salsa, and black beans.

- Lunch: Your lunch on a chilly Thursday will include Quinoa, veggie and feta salad.

- Dinner: Mouthwatering grilled fish with roasted sweet potatoes and broccoli top-up.

Friday

- Breakfast: Your weekend has you covered with tofu and vegetable frittata.

- Lunch: includes a large salad with a top-up of grilled shrimp.

- Dinner: Enjoy roasted portobello fajitas.

Saturday

- Breakfast: You can try this blackberry, kale, cashew butter, with a coconut protein smoothie.

- Lunch: make do with vegetables, avocado, and brown rice sushi with an accompaniment of seaweed salad.

- Dinner: Your weekend dinner ought to be simple and enjoyable when you eat a healthy diet of eggplant lasagna made with cheese and a large green salad.

Sunday

- Breakfast: your Sunday breakfast can include a delicious and straightforward vegetable omelet made with eggs.

- Lunch: Sumptuous meal of roasted vegetable and tahini quinoa bowl.

- Dinner: YourSunday dinner can be black bean burgers served with a large salad and sliced avocado.

It is now evident that whole-foods, plant-based diet aims to keep animal products at a minimum. However, many people on WFPB diets usually eat more or fewer animal products, which also depend entirely on their specific dietary needs, goals, or preferences.

The Bottom Line

This kind of diet is one way of eating healthy, elevating the status of different plant-based diets on the forefront, while cutting down on unhealthy meals, including added sugars and refined grains.

Plant-based diets have been linked directly to a myriad of health benefits, including a reduction in the risk of heart disease, certain types of cancers, obesity, diabetes, and a decline in our cognitive abilities. Additionally, it is worthy to transition to a more plant-based diet for our good. Irrespective of the kinds of whole-foods, a plant-based diet, which you have chosen, one thing for sure is that you are bound to lead a healthy life in the end.

What Are the Scientific Benefits of Following a Plant-Based Diet?

All over the United States of America, dietary issues have become the primary precursor for early death. This is because, on ordinary occasions, a standard American diet has very high concentrations of saturated and unprocessed fats, including sodium, and processed meat, which puts your health at a significant disadvantage when it comes to leading healthier and longer lives.

On the other side of the coin, a diet that seeks to promote whole foods and plant-based ingredients comes with numerous benefits. It can reduce the likelihood and exposure to risks generally associated with chronic illnesses. Thus, when you adhere to such diets, you also minimize over-dependence on medication, lower the exposure to risks of obesity, and high blood pressure. A plant-based diet can even help manage and keep at arm's length some type 2 diabetes and heart diseases.

A plant-based diet can also be beneficial when it comes to weight management, only if you follow it strictly. Most people who adhere to plant-based foods have reported a tremendous change in their lives in terms of energy and resilience. To realize considerable amounts of success in this matter, first of all, make a shopping list on your preferences including beans, and plant-based proteins, to pave the way for other options, which might lead you to live a healthy life.

Sticking To A Plant-Based Diet

You cannot achieve your set targets by merely adhering to a plant-based diet. It will also require you to become attentive to the kind of food you're eating. Whether it's at home or out in a restaurant, simply because in today's world, you have many outlets to sell unhealthy foods, supposedly as a plant-based item. Such types of items would include french fries and potato chips. Therefore, constant consumption of unhealthy plant-based food can expose you to the dangers of increased weight as well as other chronic conditions such as heart disease.

One notable aspect of a plant-based diet is that you need to be aware - before transitioning - is that during the initial stages, you might witness some changes in your bowel movement in that you might start to be constipated or have diarrhea. This is created because many of the foods on a plant-based diet have tons of fiber, which bring your bowel movements to be more healthy.

Moreover, for a better transition, you need to incorporate plant-based foods gradually into your meal base to give your body enough time to respond and adjust accordingly. While in the process, be sure you maintain your fluid intake - during the process itself and after transitioning.

Adopting a Whole Foods, The Plant-Based Diet is good for the planet:

It's not only beneficial to your health when you transition into a plant-based menu; scientists and environmental conservatives have also found that it helps to protect your environment as well. Those who strictly observe these types of meals tend a more significant way not to harm the environment in any manner.

This is because the adoption and maintenance of eating healthy plant meals help keep the emission of greenhouse gases at a minimum. Also kept in check are there such factors leading to environmental degradation such as global warming, will also be at a minimum. Some studies conducted by scientists and environmental lobbyists suggests that the most significant aspects of benefits to the environment came from eating plant-based meals, and the least amount of foods derived from animals. The observations cut across various plant-based products such as vegetarian and vegan diets.

How to get the most out of your plant-based meal plan?

Planning your meal is one of the best methods for maintaining your calories and eating healthy. It can also present you with some of the best ideas on how to cut on unhealthy food, prompting your family members to eat healthy as well. This is an essential fact worth mentioning, and as much as it is true, it is very complicated at the same time in numerous ways. This concept, apart from being challenging, it can be very tedious.

Nonetheless, we have many types of plant-based meal plans in this modern era, which can be very handy, these modern-day basics have made it easy for anyone keen on a healthy diet to comfortably choose what they want to eat, without any hassle. The right approach will thus guide you successfully when you have decided to embark on your meal planning journey. Apart from this, it enhances your creativity to a certain extent by coming up with hitherto unknown recipes to boot.

After you have achieved your goal of eating healthy, you might find yourself inspiring other people on the benefits of healthy living. It will be a plus for you as you will have aligned yourself to the rigorous programs that also comes with the discipline of preparing a plant-based whole meal in the long run. Practice makes perfect, and the best way in which you can engage yourself fully in the concept of a plant-based diet is to practice consistently on how to prepare such meals. In this manner, you will know the kinds of ingredients to go for on your shopping list. This will also help you come with a tangible budget when shopping for your cooking requirements. It will also make it easy for you to transition with much ease into a vegan diet.

Plant-based diets will make you keep it simple and exciting as you will only have eyes for the foods that you love most, and when the time for shopping comes, you can choose wisely your ingredients from the grocery section at your local supermarket outlet or grocery store. In the end, you will have stocked up your kitchen shelves with some of the most delicious plant-based meals and snacks as well. When you are still in learning mode, you need to stick to simple to make recipes, as you graduate to the more complex ones with time. With suck kind of learning, you can become an expert in plant-based culinary in your home, much to the delight of your family members, friends, and the extended family.

Another underlying benefit is that your delicious menu will also have the right quantities of ingredients to boot. Such an enviable experience is enough to place you at the pinnacle when it comes to catering for your various needs and those of your family successfully. Especially when coming up with a weekly or monthly budget for your home. Thus, with the right diet program at your disposal, you can be able to correctly discern the stipulated amounts of meals at the same time, saving time by planning your meals way in advance. The correct attitude will come in handy when it comes to coming up and implementing the right cooking style.

You are your boss here, hence at liberty to tinker about with any recipe in line with your taste and preferences. You can also choose to make them old fashioned or modern. The experience will also make you remember each step of the way, only topping up where necessary, with strictly and reliable, nutritious meals. There is no better time to start your journey than now. Do not be afraid to venture into the unknown, for it is only through trying that we can succeed in our undertakings. You can also explore several avenues for more ideas such as food blogs, magazines, among others. You can even venture out to one of your favorite restaurants and see what they have to offer and compare it to what you are capable of. This is the best way to learn how to prepare plant-based meals.

Why do you want to eat plant-based?

We have numerous nutritional facts on matters regarding plant-based diets. The question you should be asking yourself is, why are you transitioning to a plant-based diet, or is it right for you to do so? Overhauling your dietary needs can be overwhelming. After all, they are old habits which may very difficult to break; they could sneak back when you're not looking. Your steps will determine your actions. These are just a few of the reasons many people will be prompted to eat healthier:

- They want to lose weight

- They want to lead healthier lives

- Their love for animal

It is up to you as to why you want to try to plant-based menu plan. Do not do it because someone else is, or do it against your will. However, you will find out what time you will most likely have evolved into a more mature and solid-state of being. Try these additional steps for success:

Step 1: Write everything down.

For you not to get overwhelmed by events, you must write every step-down, as it will act as the focal point for everything regarding your plant-based meals. Jot all your reasons down and keep it somewhere where it can be accessed daily. It can either be a note stuck on the refrigerator's door, or an alert on your phone. The bottom line here is to go for what works best for you, which can be observed with much ease, something worth every time you are tempted to go back to your old ways.

Step 2. Start small but have a bigger picture in mind.

It is very satisfying when you embark on fulfilling your goals of eating healthy. What you should strive to maintain your r focus and not to feel frightened by the transition prospects. Take the process in your stride and stroll through it, no matter how hard, one day at a time and you will have succeeded before you realize it. While some people won't find any hurdles when transitioning, quite a number will find it a bit overwhelming.

Step 3: You can eat one plant-based meal a day for a period of 11 days consecutively.

Even though it seems very impossible, it can be achieved. You can try eating one plant-based meal on a daily basis for about eleven days, and then gauge if there is any significant change in your health. You might end up losing some considerable weight. However, you will also end up feeling more energetic, better sleep, and easy bowel movement. Plant-based meals will also help your body to fight the myriad of diseases, which might try to slow you down.

Step 4: Drink water in place of Sugary Drinks

You can drink water instead of soda, or any other sugary drinks. This is because with water, it very easy for you to tone down on those calories that you do not need in your diet. According to experts, you do not have to drink water alone. You can also include a variety of fruits in your diet as well. Vegetables also contain much water necessary for bodily functions. Keeping you full and hydrated at the same time. Meals such as strawberries and eggplant have approximately 90-99% water, another option to keep your body healthy and hydrated.

You Are What You Eat!

Most people believe that among the most challenging tasks concerning preparing a meal is how to come up with the right quantities for eating. Well, this can be true, especially for those who want to eat healthy by preparing their meals. Hence, it is imperative for people to generally watch what they eat to keep their weight in check, which may lead to many complications in the future. And concerning this, any meal preparation requires different recipes and portions to prepare.  It is, therefore, imperative to prepare these meals for family members for them to benefit from all the nutritional needs. That is why you must consider the right quantities before cooking and serving you and your family members. Having this mind, you can now fix the right amount of meals to prepare, and at what time, you are supposed to eat this meal.  This is vital for anyone conscious of their weight. Plant-based meals will also enable you to strictly follow the set guidelines when it comes to healthy eating and making recipes for such meals. Having a sensible plant-based meal plan will also ensure that you place clear boundaries and targets when cooking.

# Chapter 3. Breakfast recipes

## 1. Blueberry Quinoa Muffins

Preparation Time: 10Minutes

Cooking Time: 10 Minutes

Servings: 2

Ingredients

1 egg

¼ cup thick Greek yogurt

¼ cup honey

¼ tablespoon butter, melted

¼ teaspoon vanilla extract

¼ cup quinoa

1/8 cup coconut flour

¼ tablespoon baking powder

¼ teaspoon nutmeg

1/8 teaspoon salt

3/4 cup blueberries

Directions:

In a large bowl combine egg, yogurt, honey, butter, and vanilla extract until smooth.

Add quinoa, coconut flour, baking powder, nutmeg, and salt and stir just until combined.  Gently fold in blueberries.

Generously spray the 2 silicone molds with non-stick spray.  Pour batter on moulds

Stack one of the filled molds on top of a trivet.  Place 4 narrow Mason jar lids on top followed by the second silicone mould.

Pour 1 cup water into the Instant pot and place the trivet and filled silicone molds inside.

Secure the lid and turn pressure release knob to a sealed position.  Cook at high pressure for 10 minutes.

When cooking is complete, use a natural release for 10 minutes and then release any remaining pressure.

Let the quinoa bites cool if needed for handling.

Using a butter knife or spoon, scrape around each quinoa bite to release it, then turn them over on to a cooling rack or plate.

Enjoy warm as is or with a side of syrup for dipping.  Also perfect for on the go.

Store extras in the refrigerator.

Delicious chilled or warmed back up from the fridge.  Freeze beautifully as well.

Nutrition:

Calories311, Total Fat 5.7g, Saturated Fat 2.2g, Cholesterol 88mg, , Sodium 208mg, Total Carbohydrate 59.3g, Dietary Fiber 3.3g, , Total Sugars 41.5g, Protein 9.4g

## 2. Mini Frittatas

Preparation Time: 10Minutes

Cooking Time: 10 Minutes

Servings: 2

Ingredients

2 eggs

¼ teaspoon salt

1/8 teaspoon pepper

½ small red potato, small diced

¼ bell pepper, small diced

¼ small onion, small diced

1/8 cup almond milk

1/8 cup feta cheese

Directions:

Add diced vegetables to on top.

Mix eggs, milk, salt, and pepper. Pour the eggs over the veggies. Then sprinkle shredded feta cheese on top.

Cover each ramekin with foil, place them on the trivet with 1 cup water on the bottom. Cook 10 minutes on High Pressure. Once done, release the pressure using the quick release method.

Remove carefully, serve and enjoy.

Nutrition:

Calories161, Total Fat 10.1g, Saturated Fat 5.9g, Cholesterol 172mg , Sodium 463mg, Total Carbohydrate 10.3g, Dietary Fiber 1.5g , Total Sugars 2.8g, Protein 8.3g

# 3. Chocolate Muffins

 Preparation Time: 10Minutes

Cooking Time: 10 Minutes

Servings: 2

Ingredients

¼ cup coconut oil

1/8 cup honey

1 egg

½  cup almond flour

1/8 cup cocoa powder

¼  teaspoon  baking soda

1/8 teaspoon baking powder

1/6 cup almond milk

1/6 cup chocolate chips

Directions:

Add melted coconut oil and honey to a large bowl and whisk to combine, until shiny and smooth.

Add the egg and whisk.

Add almond flour, baking soda, baking powder, and cocoa powder. Whisk to combine.

Add almond milk and whisk to combine.

Stir in chocolate chips.

Spray a pressure cooker egg mold with baking spray and fill in the molds 3/4 with the muffin batter.

Add 1 1/2 cups of water to the Instant Pot and place the trivet inside.

Place the uncovered mold on top of the trivet.

Lock the lid and seal the valve.

Cook on High Pressure for 12 minutes followed by a 10-minute Natural Pressure Release.

Carefully open the lid, remove the mold.

Let it cool a bit and remove the muffins.

Sprinkle with powdered sugar and top with strawberry jam before serving if desired.

Nutrition:

Calories404, Total Fat 27.5g, Saturated Fat 10.7g,Cholesterol 85mg, Sodium 206mg, Total Carbohydrate 36.2g, Dietary Fiber 5.6g, , Total Sugars 26.5g , Protein 11.3g

# 4. Pumpkin Chocolate Chip Quinoa Muffins

Preparation Time: 10Minutes

Cooking Time: 10 Minutes

Servings: 2

Ingredients

1 egg

¼ cup canned pumpkin puree

2 tablespoons honey

¼ tablespoon coconut oil, melted

¼ teaspoon vanilla extract

¼ cup cooked quinoa

1/8 cup coconut flour

1 tablespoon baking powder

2 teaspoons pumpkin pie spice

1/4 teaspoon salt

1/3 cup mini chocolate chips

Directions:

In a large bowl whisk eggs, pumpkin puree, honey, coconut oil, and vanilla extract until smooth.

Add quinoa, coconut flour, baking powder, salt, and chocolate chips then stir just until combined.

Generously spray the 2 silicone molds with non-stick spray. Using an ice cream scoop : about 1/4 cup), divide the batter into the molds.

Stack one of the filled molds on top of a trivet. Pour 1 cup water into the pressure cooker pot and place the trivet and filled silicone molds inside.

Secure the lid and turn pressure release knob to a sealed position. Cook at high pressure for 10 minutes. When cooking is complete, use a natural release for 10 minutes and then release any remaining pressure.

Let the muffins cool if needed for handling.

Enjoy warm, as is, with a side of maple syrup, or this amazing chocolate syrup for dipping.  Also perfect for on the go.

Store extras in the refrigerator.  Delicious chilled or warmed up.

Nutrition:

Calories234, Total Fat 6.4g, Saturated Fat 3g, Cholesterol 82mg , Sodium 349mg, Total Carbohydrate 41.2g, Dietary Fiber 3.2g , Total Sugars 19.9g, Protein 6.6g

# 5. Baked Eggs with Creamy Collard Greens.

Preparation Time: 05Minutes

Cooking Time: 20 Minutes

Servings: 2

Ingredients

2 tablespoons avocado oil

½ tablespoon chopped onion

½ cup cottage cheese crumbled

½ cup collard greens

1 tablespoon coconut cream

Salt

Freshly ground black pepper

2 eggs

Chopped fresh Basil

Directions:

Select Sauté on the Instant Pot and heat 1 tablespoon of the avocado oil. Add the onion and cook, stirring occasionally, until just softened, about 1 minute. Add the cottage cheese and cook, stirring occasionally, for 2 minutes. Add the remaining avocado oil and the collard greens and cook until the greens is wilted, about 5 minutes. Add the coconut cream and 1/2 teaspoon salt and cook until most of the liquid has been reduced, about 15 minutes. Add 1/4 teaspoon pepper and taste, adjusting seasoning as desired.

Press the Cancel button to reset the program. Make two wells in the collard greens and carefully crack one egg into each well. Lock the lid in place and turn the valve to Sealing. Press the Pressure Cook button and set the cook time for 1 minute at low pressure.

Turn the valve to Venting to quick-release the steam. When the steam stops, carefully remove the lid. Transfer each egg on a bed of collard greens to a plate, top with basil, if using, and more pepper, and serve.

Nutrition:

Calories144, Total Fat 8.6g, Saturated Fat 3.7g, Cholesterol 166mg , Sodium 372mg, Total Carbohydrate 4g , Dietary Fiber 1.3g , Total Sugars 2.3g, Protein 13.3g

## 6. Ananas Quinoa

Preparation Time: 05Minutes

Cooking Time: 05 Minutes

Servings: 2

Ingredients

½ tablespoon melted butter

1 cup soy milk

½ cup pineapple juice

½ cup quinoa

½ cup fresh pineapple diced

Raspberries

Directions:

Pour butter, soy milk, pineapple juice and quinoa into Instant Pot in that order. Swirl to make sure all quinoa are submerged.

Secure the lid, making sure the vent is closed.

Using the display panel select the MANUAL function. Use the + /- keys and program the Instant Pot for 5 minutes.

When the time is up, let the pressure release naturally until the pin drops : about 15 minutes).

Stir in pineapple. Serve with raspberries.

Nutrition:

Calories300, Total Fat 7.7g, Saturated Fat 2.4g, Cholesterol 8mg , Sodium 89mg, Total Carbohydrate 47.6g, Dietary Fiber 4.7g , Total Sugars 14.1g, Protein 10.6g

# 7. Blueberries Coconut Milk Yogurt

Preparation Time: 05Minutes

Cooking Time: 14hr

Servings: 2

Ingredients

2 cups plain, sweetened coconut milk

1-1/2 tablespoon plain, dairy-free yogurt : soy, cashew, or almond

1 teaspoon vanilla extract

1 pint fresh blueberries

1 tablespoon cashew roughly chopped

2 tablespoons maple syrup

Directions:

Add the coconut milk and yogurt to the inner pot. Stir well.

Cover and lock the lid, but leave the steam release handle in the venting position. Select Yogurt and set the cook time for 14 hours. When the cook time is complete, remove the lid and stir in the vanilla extract.

Allow the yogurt to cool slightly, and then transfer to a large, seal-able glass jar, and seal tightly. Place in the refrigerator to chill and thicken for a minimum of 4 hours.

To serve, transfer the chilled yogurt to serving bowls. Top each serving with 1/2 cup blueberries and chopped cashews, and then drizzle maple syrup over top.

Nutrition:

Calories758, Total Fat 60.3g, Saturated Fat 51.2g, Cholesterol 0mg , Sodium 44mg, Total Carbohydrate 57.9g, Dietary Fiber 10.3g , Total Sugars 40.4g, Protein 8.2g

## 8. Slow Cook Barley with Apples

Preparation Time: 05Minutes

Cooking Time: 6hr

Servings: 2

Ingredients

½ cup apple diced

1 teaspoon butter

½  cup barley

2 cups Water

2 tablespoons maple syrup

Pinch salt

1/8 teaspoon cinnamon ground

½ cup soy milk light,

Walnut toasted, optional garnishing

Apple diced garnishing

Directions:

Coat the inner pot of the Instant Pot with butter. Combine apple, barley, cinnamon, maple syrup, water, soy milk and salt in inner pot.

Close and lock the lid of the Instant Pot. Turn the steam release handle to "Venting" position. Press [Slow Cook], and use [Adjust] to select "Less" mode. Press [-] or [+] to choose 6 hours cook time.

Stir well before serving. Garnish with toasted walnuts and additional diced apple, if desired. Enjoy!

Nutrition:

Calories328, Total Fat 2.2g, Saturated Fat 0.4g , Cholesterol 0mg , Sodium 123mg, Total Carbohydrate 73.2g, Dietary Fiber 13.4g, Total Sugars 31.7g , Protein 7.8g

## 9. Cottage cheese Stuffed Avocado

Preparation Time: 05Minutes

Cooking Time: 6hr

Servings: 2

Ingredients

1 large ripe avocado

½  cup Cottage cheese grated

Sea salt and black pepper, to taste

¼ cup feta Cheese, shredded

Leek , green parts only, sliced thin

Directions:

Cut avocados in half lengthwise and remove the pits. Use a spoon to carefully remove some of the avocado flesh around the pit to create more space for the filling.

Place the avocado halves into the steaming basket.

Add 1 cup of water to the Instant Pot. Lower the steaming basket with the avocados into the pressure cooker.

Scrambled cottage cheese and then carefully transfer the cottage cheese into one of the prepared avocado halves.

Repeat this process with the remaining avocado Season each with salt and black pepper, to taste.

Top each avocado half with shredded feta and leek greens.

Place the lid on the Instant Pot and lock it in place. Make sure that the vent is sealed. Cook on "Manual/High" for 4 minutes.

Once done cooking quick release the pressure before unlocking the lid.

Remove the avocados from the Instant pot Serve immediately. Enjoy!

Nutrition:

Calories300, Total Fat 22.9g, Saturated Fat 5.9g, Cholesterol 11mg , Sodium 395mg, Total Carbohydrate 14.6g, Dietary Fiber 7.2g , Total Sugars 2.7g, Protein 11.7g

# 10. Veggie Quiche

Preparation Time: 05Minutes

Cooking Time: 30 Minutes

Servings: 2

Ingredients

2 large eggs

1/8 cup coconut milk

1/8 cup coconut flour

1/8 teaspoon salt

 1/8 teaspoon pepper

½ large red pepper, chopped

¼ cup tomatoes, sliced or chopped

½ leek, chopped

2 tablespoon shredded goat cheese

¼ cup zucchini

¼ cup pumpkin

Directions:

Put trivet in the bottom of the Instant Pot. Add 1 cup of water.

In a large bowl, whisk eggs, coconut milk, coconut flour, salt and pepper. Add veggies and cheese until it's combined.

Pour the mixture into a bowl that will fit inside the Instant Pot bowl. Cover the bowl with aluminium foil and put the bowl on top of the trivet inside the Instant Pot.

Lock the Instant Pot lid. Select High Pressure and cook time of 30 minutes.

When timer beeps, let the Instant Pot sit and release pressure for 10 minutes.

Take the lid of the Instant Pot off, lift the bowl up using the sling and take off the aluminium foil.

Sprinkle the top of the quiche with the remaining 1/2 cup cheese, replace the aluminium foil and let sit until the cheese melts, about two minutes.

Serve!

Nutrition:

Calories278, Total Fat 19.1g, Saturated Fat 11.9g, Cholesterol 216mg , Sodium 329mg, Total Carbohydrate 11.6g, Dietary Fiber 2.8g , Total Sugars 5.8g, Protein 16.8g

# 11. Nutmeg Banana Quinoa

Preparation Time: 10Minutes

Cooking Time: 05 Minutes

Servings: 2

Ingredients

1 cup quinoa

1 cup soy milk

1 cup water

2 bananas

1 teaspoon nutmeg

1 tablespoon honey

Directions:

Add in the quinoa, soy milk and water in instant pot.

Slice up 1 of the bananas and add it into the Instant pot. Add in nutmeg and honey. Stir.

Set the manual button to 5 minutes. Once the timer beeps let the pressure release naturally for 10 minutes and then carefully release the rest of the pressure. Be careful though since grains can really get foamy.

Stir the quinoa and scoop into bowls. Slice the second banana and add fresh slices to the top of each bowl.

Nutrition:

Calories522, Total Fat 8.1g, Saturated Fat 1.3g, Cholesterol 0mg , Sodium 72mg, Total Carbohydrate 98.4g, Dietary Fiber 10g , Total Sugars 28.3g , Protein 17.4g

## 12. Creamy Masala Millet

Preparation Time: 10Minutes

Cooking Time: 05 Minutes

Servings: 2

Ingredients

1 cup Millet

1-1/2 cups water

½ cup heavy cream

1 tablespoon tomato paste

½ teaspoon honey

½ teaspoon ginger powder

½ teaspoon Garam masala

½ teaspoon turmeric

½ teaspoon coriander powder

1/8 teaspoon dried fenugreek leaves

¼ teaspoon chili powder

¼ teaspoon salt

Directions:

Combine all the Ingredients in the Instant Pot liner. Give it a quick stir and close the lid.

Set the valve on the "Sealed" position and pressure cook for 5 minutes. Let the pressure release naturally : about 5 minutesbefore opening the lid. Stir again using a spoon just to combine.

Divide into serving bowls topping with your choice.

Nutrition:

Calories499, Total Fat 15.5g, Saturated Fat 7.7g, Cholesterol 41mg , Sodium 339mg, Total Carbohydrate 77.6g, Dietary Fiber 9.2g, Total Sugars 2.5g, Protein 12.2g

## 13. Butternut Squash Breakfast Bowls

Preparation Time: 10Minutes

Cooking Time: 05 Minutes

Servings: 2

Ingredients

1 whole butternut squash, cut in half lengthwise and seeds removed

1 cup vanilla yogurt of choice

1  tablespoons raw peanut butter

2 teaspoons honey

1/4 teaspoon ground nutmeg

Sprinkle of hemp seeds or chia seeds

Directions:

Add 1/2 cup water to your Instant Pot and place the steamer basket inside. Place the cut and seeded butternut squash flesh side up in the Instant Pot. You can sprinkle with a little salt if desired. Secure the lid and make sure the pressure valve is set to sealing.

Set to Manual : high pressurefor 5 minutes. When cooking is complete you can either let it come to pressure naturally or perform a quick release if you are in a hurry.

To serve, make sure the butternut squash is warm or hot. Then, divide the yogurt container between the two cooked halves in the "well" of the butternut squash.

Drizzle peanut butter and honey on top. Sprinkle with nutmeg and hemp seeds.

You may want to add an optional sprinkle of salt if you didn't use salt when cooking the butternut squash to help bring out the flavours.

Serve with a spoon and be sure to get a little bit of each ingredient in every bite for the optimal experience.

Nutrition:

Calories112, Total Fat 5.1g, Saturated Fat 0.8g, Cholesterol 2mg , Sodium 45mg, Total Carbohydrate 15.1g, Dietary Fiber 3.1g , Total Sugars 6.8g, Protein 4.5g

# 14. Carrot Cake Quinoa

Preparation Time: 05Minutes

Cooking Time: 30 Minutes

Servings: 2

Ingredients

1/2 cup quinoa

1 cup water

½ cup unsweetened almond milk

1 medium carrots, grated

1 tablespoon golden raisins

1 tablespoon honey

½ teaspoon nutmeg

½ teaspoon salt

½ cup almond  for serving

Directions:

Place the quinoa, water, almond milk, carrot, golden raisins, honey, nutmeg, and salt in your Instant Pot. Stir gently to combine.

Twist the lid to lock and make sure the pressure valve is closed. Set your Instant Pot to High Pressure and adjust the timer for 10 minutes.

When the cooking time is up, turn off your Instant Pot and allow the pressure to come down naturally. This should take between 10 and 15 minutes. Eliminate any remaining pressure by flipping the quick release valve before unlocking the lid.

Stir the quinoa and adjust sweetness to taste; it will thicken a bit as it cools.

Divide the oatmeal between two bowls and garnish with chopped almond.

Nutrition:

Calories365, Total Fat 15.6g, Saturated Fat 1.4g, Cholesterol 0mg , Sodium 654mg, Total Carbohydrate 48.4g, Dietary Fiber 7.3g , Total Sugars 14g, Protein 11.7g

## 15. Broccoli Frittata with Peppers

Preparation Time: 10Minutes

Cooking Time: 30 Minutes

Servings: 2

Ingredients

½ cup sweet potato sliced

1 cup broccoli

2 eggs

1 cup coconut milk

1 teaspoon butter

1 cup shredded feta cheese

½ teaspoon Salt

¼ teaspoon ground pepper

Directions:

Grease a 6 x 3 pan. Arrange the sliced sweet potato in the bottom of the pan.

Cover with the broccoli. In a mixing bowl whisk together the eggs, butter, coconut milk, salt, and pepper. Stir In shredded cheese.

Pour the egg mixture on top of your broccoli and sweet potato and cover with foil or a silicone lid.

In the inner liner of your instant pot, place 2 cups of water.

Place a steamer rack on top of this.

Place the covered pan on the steamer rack.

Cook on high pressure for 20 minutes. Allow it to release pressure naturally for 10 minutes, and then release all remaining pressure.

Let it sit for 5-10 minutes. Using a knife, gently loosen the sides of your wondrous creation.

Serve and enjoy.

Nutrition:

Calories 477 , Total Fat 36.8g, Saturated Fat 26.5g, Cholesterol 235mg , Sodium 1536mg, Total Carbohydrate 20.3g, Dietary Fiber 4.2g , Total Sugars 9.4g, Protein 19.9g

## 16. Quinoa Burrito Bowls

Preparation Time: 10 minutes

Cooking Time: 26 minutes

Servings: 4

Ingredients:

1 cup quinoa, rinsed

1 1/2 cups cooked black beans

1/2 of medium red onion, peeled and diced

1 medium bell pepper, cored and diced

1 cup tomato salsa, and more for serving

Directions:

Switch on the instant pot, grease the inner pot with 1 teaspoon olive oil, press the sauté/simmer button, then adjust cooking time to 5 minutes and let preheat.

Add onion and pepper and cook for 8 minutes or until softened, then season with 1/2 teaspoon salt and 1 teaspoon ground cumin and cook for 1 minute or until fragrant.

Add quinoa and beans, then pour in salsa and 1 cup water, stir until mixed and press the cancel button.

Secure instant pot with its lid in the sealed position, then press the rice button, adjust cooking time to 12 minutes, select low-pressure cooking and let cook until instant pot buzz.

Instant pot will take 10 minutes or more to build pressure, and when it buzzes, press the cancel button and do natural pressure release for 10 minutes or more until pressure knob drops down.

Then carefully open the instant pot, fluff quinoa with a fork and ladle into bowls.

Serve with guacamole, salsa, and lemon wedges.

Nutrition:

Calories 657.7 , Carbohydrates 95 g , Fats 17.4 g , Protein: 34.1 g

## 17. Cilantro Lime Quinoa

Preparation Time: 10 minutes

Cooking Time: 5 minutes

Servings: 4

Ingredients:

1 1/2 cups quinoa

4-ounce green chilies

1/2 of white onion, peeled and chopped

1/2 bunch, cilantro

1 1/2 cups vegetable broth

Directions:

Place onions in a food processor, add chilies and cilantro and pulse for 1 minute or until smooth.

Switch on the instant pot, tip the onion mixture into the inner pot, season with 1 teaspoon salt and ½ teaspoon black pepper and stir until mixed.

Secure instant pot with its lid in the sealed position, then press the manual button, adjust cooking time to 5 minutes, select high-pressure cooking and let cook until instant pot buzz.

Instant pot will take 10 minutes or more to build pressure, and when it buzzes, press the cancel button and do natural pressure release for 10 minutes or more until pressure knob drops down.

Then carefully open the instant pot, fluff the quinoa and ladle into bowls.

Drizzle with lime juice and serve.

Nutrition:

Calories 550 , Carbohydrates 66 g , Fats 25 g , Protein 17 g

# 18. Pumpkin Coffeecake Oatmeal

Preparation Time: 10 minutes

Cooking Time: 3 minutes

Servings: 6

Ingredients:

1 1/2 cups oats, steel-cut

2 teaspoons cinnamon

1 teaspoon allspice

1 teaspoon vanilla extract, unsweetened

1 1/2 cups pumpkin puree

Directions:

Switch on the instant pot, place all the ingredients in the inner pot, pour in 4 1/2 cups water and stir until mixed.

Secure instant pot with its lid in the sealed position, then press the manual button, adjust cooking time to 3 minutes, select high-pressure cooking and let cook until instant pot buzz.

When instant pot buzzes, press the cancel button and do natural pressure release for 10 minutes or more until pressure knob drops down.

Then carefully open the instant pot, stir the oats and serve straight away.

Nutrition:

Calories 254, Carbohydrates 45 g , Fats 5 g , Protein 7 g

## 19. Breakfast Stuffed Sweet Potatoes

Preparation Time: 10 minutes

Cooking Time: 15 minutes

Servings: 4

Ingredients:

2 tablespoons blueberries, fresh

1 medium sweet potato

1 tablespoon chopped pecans

1 tablespoon maple syrup

1 tablespoon almond butter

Directions:

Switch on the instant pot, pour in 1 cup water, insert steamer basket and place sweet potatoes on it.

Secure instant pot with its lid in the sealed position, then press the manual button, adjust cooking time to 15 minutes, select high-pressure cooking and let cook until instant pot buzz.

Instant pot will take 10 minutes or more to build pressure, and when it buzzes, press the cancel button and do natural pressure release for 10 minutes or more until pressure knob drops down.

Carefully open the instant pot, take out the sweet potatoes, and let rest until cool enough to handle.

Then cut the sweet potato, use a fork to mash its flesh and then drizzle with butter and maple syrup.

Sprinkle potatoes with berries and pecans and serve.

Nutrition:

Calories 369 , Carbohydrates 50 g , Fats 17 g , Protein 7 g

# 20. Breakfast Potatoes

Preparation Time: 10 minutes

Cooking Time: 35 minutes

Servings: 5

Ingredients:

6 medium potatoes, peeled and ½-inch cubed

1 medium white onion, peeled and ½-inch cubed

1 medium green bell pepper, ½-inch cubed

3/4 cup vegetable broth

Directions:

Switch on the instant pot, add 3 tablespoons coconut oil in the inner pot, press the sauté/simmer button, then adjust cooking time to 5 minutes and let preheat.

Then add potatoes and cook for 3 minutes or until sauté.

Sprinkle potatoes with ¾ teaspoon salt, 1/3 teaspoon black pepper, ¼ teaspoon paprika and 1 tablespoon nutritional yeast, cook for 4 minutes and then press the cancel button.

Secure instant pot with its lid in the sealed position, then press the manual button, adjust cooking time to 1 minute, select high-pressure cooking and let cook until instant pot buzz.

Instant pot will take 10 minutes or more to build pressure, and when it buzzes, press the cancel button and do quick pressure release until pressure knob drops down.

Carefully open the instant pot, gently stir the potatoes, then transfer into a bowl and let refrigerate until cooked.

Then place a skillet pan over medium heat, grease with oil and when hot, add onion and pepper and cook for 10 minutes or until softened.

Transfer vegetables to a plate, add potatoes into the pan and cook for 10 to 15 minutes or until potatoes are crispy and nicely browned.

Return vegetables into the pan, stir well and cook for 1 minute or until thoroughly heated.

Serve immediately.

Nutrition:

Calories 157  , Carbohydrates 30 g , Fats 2.5 g , Protein 4.6 g

# 21. Burritos

Preparation Time: 10 minutes

Cooking Time: 32 minutes

Servings: 6

Ingredients:

15-ounces cooked black beans

1 1/2 cups brown rice, uncooked

1 cup chopped kale

1 medium red bell pepper, diced

12-ounce tomato salsa

Directions:

Switch on the instant pot, grease the inner pot with 3 tablespoons oil, press the sauté/simmer button, then adjust cooking time to 5 minutes and let preheat.

Add bell pepper and 1 ½ teaspoon garlic, cook for 3 minutes, then add remaining ingredients for the burrito filling, season with 1 teaspoon salt, 2 teaspoon red chili powder, 1 teaspoon paprika, 1 teaspoon cumin and stir until mixed.

Pour in 2 cups water, then press the cancel button, secure instant pot with its lid in the sealed position, press the manual button, adjust cooking time to 24 minutes, select high-pressure cooking and let cook until instant pot buzz.

Instant pot will take 10 minutes or more to build pressure, and when it buzzes, press the cancel button and do natural pressure release for 10 minutes or more until pressure knob drops down.

Then carefully open the instant pot, stir the mixture and taste to adjust seasoning.

Spoon the mixture evenly on tortillas, top with lettuce, avocado, and cheese and serve with salsa.

Nutrition:

Calories 491  , Carbohydrates 70 g , Fats 16 g , Protein 21 g

## 22. Chocolate Banana Cake

Preparation Time: 10 minutes

Cooking Time: 30 minutes

Servings: 6

Ingredients:

For the cake:

1 ½ cups of water

3 medium ripe bananas, peeled

½ cup coconut sugar

½ cup beets sugar

1 tsp vanilla extract

¼ cup coconut cream

2 ¼ tsp active dry yeast

2 cups all-purpose flour, sifted

1 tsp baking powder

1 tsp baking soda

½ tsp salt

2 tsp unsweetened cocoa powder

Poppy seeds for topping

For the vanilla-icing glaze:

¼ cup coconut milk

1 tsp vanilla extract

2 tbsp coconut sugar

2 tbsp vegan butter, melted

Directions:

Open the lid of the instant pot, pour in the water, and fit a trivet with handles in the pot.

Grease a 7-inch Bundt pan with non-stick cooking spray and set aside.

In a small bowl, put the bananas and mash with a fork until a paste-like consistency form. Set aside.

In another bowl, whisk the coconut sugar, beet sugar, vanilla extract, and coconut cream until creamy. Add and stir in the banana until mixed.

In a separate bowl, combine the dry yeast, flour, baking powder, baking soda, and cocoa powder until evenly mixed.

Add the dry ingredients to the banana mixture and mix until well combined.

Pour the mixture into the cake pan and place the pan on the trivet in the pot.

Close the lid of the pot, secure the pressure valve, and select Manual mode on high pressure. Set the timer for 30 minutes.

While the bread bakes, make the vanilla-icing glaze. In a bowl, add the coconut milk, vanilla extract, coconut sugar, vegan butter, and whisk the ingredients until a smooth, runny cream forms. Set aside.

When the pot's timer beeps, perform a natural pressure release until all the steam escapes, and then carefully open the lid.

Hold the handles of the trivet with napkins and lift out of the pot with the bread pan.

Remove the bread onto a plate, allow cooling for 5 minutes, and drizzle the vanilla icing glaze all over on top. Sprinkle with some poppy seeds and cut the bread into slices.

Serve immediately as a breakfast compliment.

Nutrition:

Calories 472, Carbohydrates 77g, Fats 13.5 g, Protein 7.8 g

## 23. Breakfast Chocolate Quinoa

Preparation Time: 4 minutes

Cooking Time: 2 minutes

Servings: 6

Ingredients:

For the quinoa:

1 1/2 cups white quinoa, rinsed

1 cup almond milk + extra for serving

½ cup coconut milk

1 tbsp unsweetened cocoa powder

2 tbsp coconut sugar + extra for topping

1/2 tsp vanilla extract

A pinch of salt

For topping:

Mixed berries

Banana slices

Chopped almonds

4 squares vegan chocolate, chopped

Directions:

Open the instant pot and pour in the quinoa, almond milk, coconut milk, cocoa powder, coconut sugar, vanilla extract, and salt. Give the ingredients a good stir with a spoon.

Close the lid of the pot, secure the pressure valve, and select Manual mode on high pressure. Set the timer to 2 minutes to cook.

Once the timer beeps, perform a natural pressure release for 10 minutes, then a quick pressure release to let out the remaining steam.

When the valve drops, carefully open the lid while tilting away from your face. Stir the quinoa and spoon the food into breakfast bowls.

Pour some almond milk on top, sprinkle with some coconut sugar as desired, and top with the berries, banana, almonds, and dark chocolate.

Nutrition:

Calories 637, Carbohydrates 76.6 g, Fats 31.7 g, Protein 14.4 g

## 24. Buttery Sweet Corn Porridge

Preparation Time: 4 minutes

Cooking Time: 2 minutes

Servings: 4

Ingredients:

For the corn porridge:

1 cup yellow cornmeal, coarse

4 cups of water

¼ cup coconut milk

2 tbsp coconut sugar

¼ tsp cinnamon powder

½ tsp vanilla extract

¼ tsp nutmeg powder

4 tbsp vegan butter

For the toppings:

Papaya slices

Raspberries

Toasted shredded coconut

Directions:

Open the instant pot and add the cornmeal, water, coconut milk, coconut sugar, cinnamon powder, vanilla extract, and nutmeg powder. Stir the ingredients with a spoon.

Close the lid of the pot, secure the pressure valve, and select Porridge mode on high pressure. Set the timer for 2 minutes.

When the timer is done, perform a natural pressure release for 10 minutes, then a quick pressure release to let out any remaining steam, and open the lid.

Add the vegan butter, stir the porridge with a spoon until the butter melts, and adjust the taste with some coconut sugar.

Dish the food into serving bowls and top with some papaya, raspberries, and sprinkle the shredded coconut on the side.

Nutrition:

Calories 311, Carbohydrates 38.9 g, Fats 15.8 g, Protein 3.4 g

## 25. Sweet Potato Hash Brown Bowls

Preparation Time: 8 minutes

Cooking Time: 23 minutes

Servings: 4

Ingredients:

1 cup water

1 ½ lb. sweet potatoes, cubed

2 tbsp vegetable oil

1 large red onion, peeled and diced

¼ sliced white mushrooms

1 red bell pepper, deseeded and diced

1 garlic clove, minced

Salt and black pepper to taste

1 tsp sweet paprika

1 tsp hot sauce

1 : 8 ozblack beans, drained and rinsed

1 tbsp freshly chopped parsley

1 tsp dried oregano

Serving:

1 avocado, pitted and chopped

Chopped parsley to garnish

Directions:

Turn on and open the instant pot; add the water into the pot.

Pour the potatoes into a steamer basket and fit the basket into the pot over the water.

Close the lid, secure the pressure valve, and select Manual mode on high pressure. Set the timer for 12 minutes.

Once the pot beeps, do a natural pressure release for 15 to 20 minutes, and then open the lid.

Carefully remove the steamer basket and set aside the potatoes to cool. Discard the water in the pot and select Sauté mode.

Pour the oil into the pot to heat and add the onion, mushrooms, and red bell pepper. Stir-fry until the vegetables have softened, 7 minutes.

Add the potatoes, garlic, salt, black pepper, paprika, hot sauce, black beans, parsley, and oregano. Stir and cook the ingredients until the flavors adequately incorporate, 4 minutes.

Adjust the taste with salt and black pepper and turn the pot off. Spoon the dish into serving bowls and garnish with avocado and parsley.

Nutrition:

Calories 256, Carbohydrates 27.8 g, Fats 15.9 g, Protein 8.5 g

## 26. Cranberry Rice Pudding

Preparation Time: 3 minutes

Cooking Time: 5 minutes

Servings: 4

Ingredients:

1 cup jasmine rice, rinsed

4 cups of coconut milk

½ tsp nutmeg powder

1 tsp vanilla extract

¼ cup maple syrup

½ cup dried cranberries

¼ cup almonds

Directions:

Open the instant pot and pour in the rice, coconut milk, nutmeg, vanilla extract, and maple syrup.

Close the lid, secure the pressure valve, and select Manual mode on high pressure. Set the timer for 5 minutes.

When done cooking, perform a natural pressure release to let out all the steam, and then carefully open the lid. Add the cranberries to the pudding and stir. Dish the pudding, scatter some almonds on top and serve warm.

Nutrition:

Calories 381, Carbohydrates 76 g, Fats 3 g, Protein 11.5 g

## 27. Maple Kiwi Oatmeal

Preparation Time: 5 minutes

Cooking Time: 3 minutes

Servings: 4

Ingredients:

For the oatmeal:

2 cups Scottish oatmeal

8 cups almond milk

½ cup maple syrup

2 tbsp vegan butter

1 tsp vanilla extract

½ tsp salt

½ tsp cinnamon powder

½ tsp nutmeg powder

For the topping:

¼ cup chopped mangoes

¼ cup chopped kiwis

A handful of toasted coconut shavings

Cinnamon powder for sprinkling

Directions:

Open the instant pot and pour in the oats, almond milk, maple syrup, vegan butter, vanilla extract, salt, cinnamon, and nutmeg. Stir the ingredients with a spoon.

Close the lid of the pot, secure the pressure valve, and select Manual mode on high pressure. Set the timer for 3 minutes.

Once the timer has ended, perform a natural pressure release for 10 minutes, then a quick pressure release until all the steam escapes, and then carefully open the lid.

Stir the oatmeal and adjust the taste with some more maple syrup as desired. Dish the oatmeal into serving bowls, top with the mangoes, kiwis, coconut shavings, and sprinkle with the cinnamon powder.

Nutrition:

Calories 443, Carbohydrates 74 g, Fats 8.1 g, Protein 20 g

## 28. Raspberry Toast Casserole

Preparation Time: 5 minutes

Cooking Time: 15 minutes

Servings: 4

Ingredients:

1 loaf vegan multigrain bread

1 cup almond milk

1 tbsp brown sugar

2 tbsp cornstarch

1 tsp vanilla extract

2 tbsp melted vegan butter

A pinch salt

¼ tsp cinnamon powder

¼ cup raspberries

Directions:

Place the bread on a chopping board and cut into 1-inch slices. Set aside.

In a bowl, whisk the almond milk, brown sugar, cornstarch, vanilla extract, vegan butter, salt, and cinnamon powder.

Turn on and open the instant pot; pour the water into the pot and fit in a trivet with handles.

In a heatproof bowl, scatter the bread slices and raspberries and pour the cornstarch mixture all over.

Cover the bowl with aluminum foil and place the bowl on the trivet.

Close the lid, secure the pressure valve, and select Manual mode on high pressure. Set the timer for 15 minutes.

When the timer beeps, perform a natural pressure release for 10 minutes, then a quick pressure release to let out the remaining steam, and carefully open the lid. Remove the bowl from the pot onto a flat surface.

Dish the casserole into plates and drizzle with some maple syrup.

Nutrition:

Calories 287, Carbohydrates 25.8 g, Fats 11.2 g, Protein 6.9 g

# 29. Mediterranean Scramble Tofu Tacos

Preparation Time: 15 minutes

Cooking Time: 10 minutes

Servings: 4

Ingredients:

For the tacos:

1 : 14 ozextra firm tofu

2 tbsp olive oil

1 small red onion, chopped

1 clove garlic, minced

1 red bell pepper, deseeded and diced

¼ tsp turmeric powder

¼ tsp sumac

Salt and black pepper to taste

½ tsp red chili flakes

3 green onions, chopped

For assembling:

8 corn tortillas

Chopped cilantro

1 large tomato, chopped

1 avocado, pitted and chopped

Hot sauce, as desired

Directions:

Wrap the tofu in paper towels and set aside to soak excess liquid for 10 minutes. After, crumble the tofu into a plate and set aside. Turn on and open the instant pot; select Sauté mode.

Pour in the olive oil to heat and add the onion, garlic, and red bell pepper. Stir-fry the vegetables until softened, 4 minutes.

Season with the turmeric, sumac, salt, black pepper, and red chili flakes. Cook for 5 minutes, stirring frequently. Stir in green onions, cook for 1 minute.

To assemble, lay the tortillas on a flat surface and share the tofu into the center of each tortilla. Top with cilantro, tomato, avocado, and hot sauce.

Nutrition:

Calories 424, Carbohydrates 34.2 g, Fats 27.5 g, Protein 15.6 g

## 30. Kale Potato Breakfast Sauté

Preparation Time: 8 minutes

Cooking Time: 17 minutes

Servings: 4

Ingredients:

1 cup water

½ lb. potatoes, rinsed and cubed

1 lb. butternut squash, diced

2 tbsp olive oil

1 medium onion, peeled and diced

1 yellow bell pepper, chopped

2 cups kale, chopped

2 cloves garlic, minced

Salt and black pepper to taste

Directions:

Turn on and open the instant pot; pour the water into the pot. Place the potatoes and butternut squash into a steamer basket and fit the basket into the pot over the water.

Close the lid, secure the pressure valve, and select Manual mode on high pressure. Set the timer for 12 minutes.

When the timer is done reading, perform a natural pressure release for 15 minutes, and then open the lid. Carefully remove the steamer basket and set the vegetables aside. Also, discard the water in the pot.

Select Sauté mode on the pot and add the oil to heat.

Pour in the onion, bell pepper and stir-fry the ingredients until softened for 3 minutes.

Stir in the potatoes, butternut squash, kale, garlic, salt, and black pepper and cook until the kale wilts and color changes to a light green color. Stir occasionally. Adjust the taste with salt and black pepper and turn the heat off.

Dish the food onto plates and serve warm with orange juice.

Nutrition:

Calories 280, Carbohydrates 38.7 g, Fats 7.1 g, Protein 5.3 g

## 31. Curried Chickpea Flour Frittata

Preparation Time: 8 minutes

Cooking Time: 15 minutes

Servings: 4

Ingredients:

2 cups chickpea flour

1 tsp baking powder

2 ½ cups of water

1 tbsp nutritional yeast

1 tsp Mexican seasoning mix

½ tsp yellow curry powder

Salt to taste

¼ tsp red chili flakes

1 red bell pepper, deseeded and chopped

1 green bell pepper, chopped

¼ cup sweet corn kernels

1 cup chopped spinach

½ cup vegan cheese, crumbled

1 ½ cups water

Directions:

In a medium bowl, mix the chickpea flour, baking powder, water, nutritional yeast, Mexican-seasoning mix, curry powder, salt, and chili flakes until evenly combined. After, fold in the bell peppers, corn kernels, and spinach.

Pour the mixture into a safe heat bowl that will fit into the instant pot, scatter some vegan cheese on top, and cover with aluminum foil.

Turn on and open the instant pot. Pour the water into the pot and fit a trivet over the pot. Place the bowl on the trivet and close the lid.

Secure the pressure valve and select Manual mode on high pressure. Set the timer for 15 minutes.

Once done reading, perform a quick pressure release, and open the lid. Carefully lift the bowl out of the pot onto a flat surface. Take off the aluminum foil and slice the frittata. Serve the frittata with arugula and tomato salad.

Nutrition:

Calories 262, Carbohydrates 34.4 g, Fats 6.8 g, Protein 15.9 g

## 32. Tropical Fruits Grits

Preparation Time: 5 minutes

Cooking Time: 10 minutes

Servings: 4

Ingredients:

For the grits:

1 ½ cups yellow cornmeal grits

2 cups of water

¾ cup almond milk + extra for topping

½ tsp salt

2 tbsp maple syrup + extra for topping

For topping:

2 kiwis, peeled and chopped

¼ cup chopped pineapples

2 bananas, sliced

4 strawberries, sliced

Directions:

Turn on and open the instant pot.

Add the cornmeal grits, water, almond milk, salt, and maple syrup. Stir the ingredients.

Close the lid, secure the pressure valve, and select Manual mode on high pressure. Set the timer for 10 minutes.

When the timer is done, perform a natural pressure release for 15 minutes, and then a quick pressure release to let out the remaining steam. Carefully open the lid.

Stir and spoon the grits into breakfast bowls, pour some almond milk on top, followed by a combination of the kiwis, pineapples, bananas, and strawberries, and then some maple syrup.

Serve the grits warm.

Nutrition:

Calories 336, Carbohydrates 75 g, Fats 1.7 g, Protein 5.3 g

## 33. Spicy Polenta and Buttered Spinach

Preparation Time: 5 minutes

Cooking Time: 26 minutes

Servings: 4

Ingredients:

For the polenta:

½ cup instant polenta

1 cup coconut milk

3 tbsp vegan butter

Salt and black pepper to taste

1 ½ cups vegan cheese

Olive oil for topping

For the buttered spinach:

3 tbsp vegan butter

2 garlic cloves, minced

1 ½ cups baby spinach

For topping:

Toasted pine nuts

Directions:

Make the buttered spinach first. Turn on, open the instant pot, and select Sauté mode.

Add the vegan butter to melt and then the garlic, stir-fry until fragrant but not brown.

Put in the spinach and cook until partially wilted about 3 to 4 minutes. Spoon the spinach onto a plate, cover with another plate, and set aside.

Turn the pot off and wipe the inner part clean with a paper towel.

Pour in the polenta, coconut milk, vegan butter, salt, and black pepper.

Close the lid, secure the pressure valve, and select Porridge mode, which will cook the food automatically for 20 minutes.

Once the timer is done, perform a natural pressure release until all the steam escapes, and carefully open the lid.

Add the vegan cheese and stir the polenta until the cheese melts. Dish the food into serving bowls. Spoon the spinach on top, drizzle with olive oil, and top with the pine nuts.

Nutrition:

Calories 370, Carbohydrates 12 g, Fats 30.9 g, Protein 14.5 g

## 34. Psyllium Flatbread

Servings: 6

Preparation Time: 10 min

Cooking Time: 25 min

Ingredients:

Goat cheese – 6 oz.

Eggs - 3

Psyllium husk powder – 6 tablespoons

Dried blueberries : frozen– 2 tablespoons

Baking powder – ½ teaspoon

Directions:

Combine the eggs and goat cheese in a bowl, mixing well.

Mix in the baking powder, blueberries and then the mix in the husk powder.

Leave aside for a minute and then transfer the mixture into a baking tray lined with parchment paper.

Bake for 25 minutes in an oven preheated to 350 degrees Fahrenheit.

Nutrition: 136 Cal, 8.5 g total fat, 2.2 g net carb., 5.3g fiber, 7 g protein.

## 35. Coconut Crepes

Servings: 2

Preparation Time: 10 min

Cooking Time: 32 min

Ingredients:

Coconut flour – 2 tablespoons

Heavy cream – 4 tablespoons

Eggs – 2

Water – ½ cup

Butter – 1 tablespoon

Salt – Just a pinch

Directions:

Add some butter over medium flame and spread.

Place the rest of the ingredients in a blender and blend until smooth.

Add 2 tablespoon of the blended batter on the pan and spread until you get a thin crepe.

Cook until it begins bubbling on the top after 3-5 minutes and then flip, cooking for an additional 30 seconds.

Add some butter again and repeat with the rest of the batter.

Nutrition: 260 Cal, 22.2 g total fat, 3.9 g net carb., 3.2g fiber, 8.2 g protein.

## 36. Chia Almond Smoothie

Servings: 1

Preparation Time: 3 min

Ingredients:

Almond milk – ½ cup

Almond butter – 2 tablespoon

Chia seeds : ground– 2 tablespoon

Coconut cream – ¼ cup

Vanilla – 1 teaspoon

Natural yoghurt : unsweetened– ½ cup

Granulated sweetener – 1 tablespoon

Directions:

Combine all the ingredients in a high speed blender.

Blend until smooth.

Nutrition: 581 Cal, 50 g total fat, 25 g carb., 12g fiber, 17 g protein.

## 37. Nut Packed Coconut Granola

Servings: 20

Preparation Time: 5 min

Cooking Time: 28 min

Ingredients:

Coconut flakes : unsweetened– ½ cup

Raw almonds : slivered– 2 cups

Raw pecans – 1 ¼ cup

Raw walnuts – 1 cup

Chia seeds – 3 tablespoon

Flax seed meal – 1 tablespoon

Cinnamon : ground– 1 ½ teaspoon

Coconut sugar – 2 tablespoon

Sea salt – ¼ teaspoon

Coconut oil – 3 tablespoon

Maple syrup – ¼ cup + 1 tablespoon

Dried blueberries – ¼ cup

Roasted sunflower seeds : unsalted– ¼ cup

Directions:

Mix together the nuts, coconut, coconut sugar, cinnamon, flax seed meal, and salt in a bowl.

Heat the coconut oil and maple syrup lightly in a saucepan over medium flame and pour it over the mixture in the bowl.

Transfer the mixture onto a baking sheet, spreading it well and bake in an oven preheated to 325 degrees Fahrenheit for 20 minutes.

Mix in the sunflower seeds and blueberries and bake at 340 degrees Fahrenheit for 5-8 minutes.

Remove and leave to cool.

Nutrition: 218 Cal, 18.5 g total fat : 3.6 g sat. fat), 24 mg sodium, 10.6 g carb., 4.7g fiber, 6.2 g protein.

## 38. Choco – Breakfast Waffles

Servings: 5

Preparation Time: 15 min

Cooking Time: 20 min

Ingredients:

Eggs : separated– 5

Coconut flour – 4 tablespoon

Cocoa : unsweetened– ¼ cup

Granulated sweetener – 3 tablespoon

Baking powder – 1 teaspoon

Vanilla – 1 teaspoon

Full-fat milk – 3 tablespoon

Butter : melted– 4 ½ oz.

Directions:

Place the egg whites in a bowl and whisk till stiff peaks are formed.

In another bowl mix together the coconut flour, egg yolks, cocoa, baking powder and sweetener.

Gradually add in the butter to the dry mix and mix well.

Mix in the milk and vanilla.

Finally, fold in the egg whites, a little at a time.

Transfer the mixture onto a baking sheet, spreading it well Place portions of the mixture into a heated waffle maker and cook until golden.

Repeat with the rest of the mixture.

Nutrition: 289 Cal, 26.6 g total fat,7g carb., 3.6g fiber, 7.2 g protein.

## 39. Pumpkin Spice Scones

Servings: 6

Preparation Time: 10 min

Cooking Time: 40 min

Ingredients:

Coconut flour – ½ cup

Salted butter – ¼ cup

Greek yoghurt – 6 tablespoon

Pumpkin puree - 6 tablespoon

Eggs – 2

Swerve – 2 tablespoon

Pumpkin pie spice – 2 teaspoon

Directions:

Mix together the coconut flour, spices and Swerve in a bowl.

Cut the butter into the flour mix until it resembles crumbs.

Mix in the pumpkin puree and yoghurt, till well combined.

Mix in the eggs, one at a time, till incorporated completely.

Scoop the mixture onto a baking tray and bake in an oven preheated to 350 degrees Fahrenheit for 40 minutes until the tops just begin to brown.

Leave to cool.

Nutrition: 137 Cal, 11 g total fat,3.7g net carb., 5.8g fiber, 6.3 g protein.

# 40. Streusel Scones

Servings: 12

Preparation Time: 15 min

Cooking Time: 20 min

Ingredients:

Almond flour – 2 cups

Baking powder – 1 teaspoon

Ground stevia leaf – ¼ teaspoon

Fresh blueberries – 1 cup

Salt – Just a pinch

Egg – 1

Almond milk – 2 tablespoons

Topping:

Egg white – 1 tablespoon

Slivered almonds – ¼ cup

Cinnamon : ground– ½ teaspoon

Stevia – Just a pinch

Directions:

Mix together all the topping ingredients in a bowl and place aside.

In another bowl, mix together the flour, stevia, salt and baking powder, whisking to combine.

Mix in the blueberries.

Mix the milk and egg in yet another bowl and pour it into the flour mix until well combined.

Shape portions of the mixture to form 12 scones and place on a cookie sheet lined with parchment paper.

Bake in an oven preheated to 375 degrees Fahrenheit for 20-22 minutes until golden.

Nutrition: 145 Cal, 11.6 g total fat : 1.3 g sat. fat), 12 mg sodium, 5.9 g carb., 2.6g fiber, 0.6 g protein.

## 41. Strawberry Choco-Protein Shake

Servings: 2

Preparation Time: 5 min

Ingredients:

Almond milk : unsweetened– 16 oz.

Heavy cream – 4 oz.

Chocolate Whey Isolate powder : from Jay Robb– 2 scoops

Strawberry syrup : sugar free– 1 tablespoon

Crushed ice – ½ cup

Directions:

Combine all the ingredients in a high speed blender.

Blend until smooth.

Nutrition: 351 Cal, 25 g total fat, 4 g carb., 2.6g fiber, 27 g protein.

## 42. Cinnamon Cauliflower Oatmeal

Servings: 6

Preparation Time: 10 min

Cooking Time: 10 min

Ingredients:

Crushed pecans : toasted– 1 cup

Flax seed – 1/3 cup

Chia seed – 1/3 cup

Cauliflower : riced– ½ cup

Coconut milk – 3 ½ cups

Cream cheese – 3 oz.

Heavy cream – ¼ cup

Butter – 3 tablespoon

Cinnamon – 1 ½ teaspoon

Maple flavor – 1 teaspoon

Vanilla – ½ teaspoon

Nutmeg – ¼ teaspoon

Allspice – ¼ teaspoon

Erythritol : powdered– 3 tablespoon

Xanthan gum – 1/8 teaspoon

Liquid stevia – 10 drops

Directions:

Heat the coconut milk in a pan over low flame and add the pecans to it.

Add the cauliflower and bring to boil.

Reduce the flame and simmer.

Mix in the spices, erythritol, stevia, chia seeds and flax seeds.

Mix in the butter, cream cheese and xanthan gum.

Nutrition: 398 Cal, 37.7 g total fat, 3.1 g net carb., 8.8 g protein.

## 43. Smoothie Bowl

Servings: 1

Preparation Time: 5 min

Ingredients:

Spinach – 1 cup

Almond milk – ½ cup

Heavy cream – 2 tablespoon

Coconut oil – 1 tablespoon

Low-carb protein powder – 1 scoop

Ice cubes - 2

Topping:

Raspberries - 4

Walnuts - 4

Chia seeds – 1 teaspoon

Shredded coconut – 1 tablespoon

Directions:

Combine all the smoothie ingredients in a blender and blend until smooth.

Transfer into a bowl and top with all the toppings.

Nutrition: 570 Cal, 35 g total fat, 4 g carb., 35 g protein.

## 44. Maple-Pecan Fat Bars

Servings: 12

Preparation Time: 10 min

Cooking Time: 30 min

Ingredients:

Pecan halves – 2 cups

Almond flour – 1 cup

Golden flaxseed meal – ½ cup

Shredded coconut : unsweetened– ½ cup

Coconut oil – ½ cup

Maple syrup – ¼ cup

Liquid stevia – ¼ teaspoon

Directions:

Toast the pecans at 350 degrees Fahrenheit in an oven for 6-7 minutes and then crush by placing in a plastic bag.

Mix together all the dry ingredients in a bowl including the crushed pecans.

Mix in the wet ingredients and make a dough that is still crumbly.

Spread the mixture onto a casserole dish and press.

Bake for 20-25 minutes.

Leave to cool at room temperature and then refrigerate for an hour.

Nutrition: 303 Cal, 30.5 g total fat, 2 g net carb., 4.9 g protein.

# 45. Macadamia Berry Granola

Servings: 8

Preparation Time: 10 min

Cooking Time: 20 min

Ingredients:

Macadamia nuts : chopped– 4 oz.

Raw almonds : sliced, chopped)– 4 oz.

Raw cacao nibs – 2 oz.

Flaked coconut : unsweetened– 1 ½ oz.

Strawberries : frozen, dried– ½ cup

Butter : melted– 2 tablespoons

Egg white : beaten– 1

Sukrin Fiber Syrup Clear – ¼ cup

Swerve Confectioners - 1 tablespoon

Salt – Just a pinch

Directions:

Toss together the nuts, cacao nibs and salt in a bowl and then mix in the butter.

Mix in the syrup and then the egg white.

Transfer the granola onto a baking sheet lined with parchment paper and spread.

Bake in an oven preheated to 325 degrees Fahrenheit for 15-25 minutes.

Leave to cool and then toss in the strawberries and coconut flakes.

Nutrition: 297Cal, 27 g total fat, 16 g carb., 11 g fiber, 6 g protein.

## 46. Cinnamon Apple Breakfast bars

Servings: 8

Preparation Time: 5 min

Cooking Time: 25 min

Ingredients:

Eggs - 4

Pecans : made into flour– 1 cup

Frozen dried apples : crumbled– ¼ cup

Coconut butter – ¼ cup

Five spice blend – 2 teaspoon

Vanilla extract – 1 teaspoon

Liquid stevia – 10 drops

Directions:

Mix together all the ingredients in a bowl.

Transfer into a greased baking pan and spread evenly.

Bake in an oven preheated to 350 degrees Fahrenheit for 25 minutes until a knife inserted comes out clean.

Nutrition: 184 Cal, 16.5 g total fat, 2.5 g carb., 2.6 g fiber, 5 g protein.

# 47. Scrambled Eggs with Pesto

Servings: 1

Preparation Time: 5 min

Cooking Time: 5 min

Ingredients:

Eggs - 3

Butter – 1 tablespoon

Green pesto – 1 tablespoon

Creamed coconut milk – 2 tablespoon

Salt to taste

Ground pepper to taste

Directions:

Beat together the eggs, salt and pepper.

Melt butter on a pan and add the eggs to it on low flame, stirring continuously until dried up.

Mix in the pesto.

Remove from the flame and mix in the coconut milk.

Nutrition: 467 Cal, 41.5 g total fat : 19.6 g sat. fat), 3.3 g carb., 0.7 g fiber, 20.4 g protein.

## 48. Breakfast Pudding

Servings: 3

Preparation Time: 5 min

Ingredients:

Coconut milk : full-fat– 1 ½ cup

Frozen raspberries – 1 cup

MCT oil – ¼ cup

Apple cider vinegar – 1 tablespoon

Vanilla extract – 1 teaspoon

Stevia – 3 drops

Chia seeds – 2 tablespoons

Fresh berries – for topping

Directions:

Combine all the ingredients in a food processor.

Blend until smooth.

Serve chilled topped with fresh berries.

Nutrition: 328 Cal, 34.2 g total fat : 30.8 g sat. fat), 8.8g carb., 3.1 g fiber, 3.2 g protein.

## 49. Mushroom & Kale Omelet

Servings: 2

Preparation Time: 15 min

Cooking Time: 15 min

Ingredients:

Eggs - 4

Butter – 1 tablespoon

Kale leaf : chopped– 1

White button mushrooms : chopped– 6

Table salt – just a dash

Cheddar cheese – 4 thin slices

Cheshire cheese – 1 thin slice

Jarlsberg Swiss cheese - 1 thin slice

Directions:

Melt the butter in a pan on low flame and sauté the mushrooms and kale in it with a pinch of salt, until softened.

Blend together the eggs, Cheshire cheese, Jarlsberg Swiss cheese, cream and one slice of Cheddar cheese in a blender.

Add the egg mixture to the pan and cook covered until firm.

Add the rest of the cheese slices and fold the omelet over.

Nutrition: 349.8 Cal, 29.2 g total fat, 432.3 mg chol., 584.6 mg sodium, 4.1 g carb., 1 g fiber, 18.2 g protein.

## 50. Garlicky Coconut Bagels

Servings: 6

Preparation Time: 5 min

Cooking Time: 15 min

Ingredients:

Eggs - 6

Butter : melted– 1/3 cup

Coconut flour : sifted– ½ cup

Guar gum – 2 teaspoons

Garlic powder – 1 ½ teaspoons

Salt – ½ teaspoon

Baking powder – ½ teaspoon

Directions:

Mix together the butter, eggs, garlic powder and salt.

Mix together the flour, gum and baking powder in another bowl.

Add the dry mixture to the wet, mixing well until no lumps are formed.

Grease a donut pan and transfer the mixture into it.

Bake for 15 minutes at 400 degrees Fahrenheit.

Leave to cool.

Nutrition: 191 Cal, 16 g total fat : 9 g sat. fat), 213 mg chol., 352.2 mg sodium, 6 g carb., 3 g fiber, 8 g protein.

## 51. Tomato Zucchini Bread

Servings: 12

Preparation Time: 10 min

Cooking Time: 50 min

Ingredients:

Eggs - 4

Salted butter : melted– ¾ cup

Almond milk : unsweetened– ½ cup

Zucchini : shredded, dried with paper towel– ½ cup

Sun dried tomatoes : chopped– 2 tablespoons

Almond flour – 2 cups

Coconut flour – ¼ cup

Baking powder – 4 teaspoon

Granulated sugar substitute – 1 teaspoon

Kosher salt – 1 ¼ teaspoon

Xanthan gum – ½ teaspoon

Dried oregano – ½ teaspoon

Dried parsley – ½ teaspoon

Garlic powder – ¼ teaspoon

Shredded Asiago cheese – ½ cup

Directions:

Mix together all the wet ingredients in a blender and blend until smooth.

Mix together all the dry ingredients in a bowl.

Add the wet mixture to the dry, mixing well until no lumps are formed.

Mix in the cheese.

Grease a loaf pan and transfer the mixture into it.

Bake for 50-60 minutes at 350 degrees Fahrenheit.

Nutrition: 262 Cal, 23 g total fat, 3 g net carb., 8 g protein.

## 52. Coconut Muesli

Servings: 15

Preparation Time: 1 min

Cooking Time: 8 min

Ingredients:

Flaked coconut : unsweetened– 1 cup

Sunflower seeds – 1 cup

Pumpkin seeds – 1 cup

Almonds : sliced– 1 cup

Pecans – ½ cup

Hemp hearts – ½ cup

Cinnamon – 2 teaspoons

Vanilla extract – ½ teaspoon

Vanilla stevia – ¼ teaspoon

Directions:

Toss together all the ingredients in a baking pan.

Bake for 7-8 minutes at 350 degrees Fahrenheit.

Leave to cool.

Serve with almond milk.

Nutrition: 200 Cal, 17.8 g total fat, 3 mg sodium, 6.1 g carb., 3.3g fiber, 6.9 g protein.

## 53. Vanilla Smoothie

Servings: 1

Preparation Time: 2 min

Ingredients:

Egg yolks - 2

Mascarpone cheese : full-fat– ½ cup

Water – ¼ cup

Ice cubes - 4

Coconut oil – 1 tablespoon

Powdered Erythritol – 1 tablespoon

Pure vanilla extract – 1 teaspoon

Directions:

Combine all the ingredients in a blender.

Blend until smooth.

Nutrition: 650 Cal, 64 g total fat,  4 g carb., 12 g protein.

# Chapter 4. Lunch recipes

## 54. Basil and Garlic Seitan Roast

Preparation Time: 5minutes

Cooking Time: 15minutes

Servings: 6

Ingredients:

3 lb seitan roast

5 cloves garlic, minced

Salt and ground black pepper to taste

1 tbsp Dijon mustard

1 tsp dried basil

2 tsp garlic powder

Directions:

Preheat the oven to 400 F and place the seitan in a baking dish.

In a small bowl, mix the minced garlic, salt, black pepper, mustard, basil, and garlic powder. Rub the mixture all over the seitan. Drizzle with the olive oil and place in the oven to bake for 10 to 15 minutes or until the seitan cooks within and brown outside.

Remove the dish from the oven, transfer the seitan onto a flat surface, and allow cooling for 5 minutes.

Slice and serve with steamed greens.

Nutrition:

Calories:224, Total Fat:20.4g, Saturated Fat:12.2g, Total Carbs:1g, Dietary Fiber:0g, Sugar:1g, Protein:9g, Sodium:556mg

## 55. Beet Greens with Tofu Chops

Preparation Time: 10minutes

Cooking Time: 20minutes

Servings: 4

Ingredients:

2 tbsp balsamic vinegar

Salt and ground black pepper to taste

2 tsp freshly pureed garlic

2 tbsp freshly chopped basil

4 : 2-inchslabs extra firm tofu

4 thyme sprigs

1 tbsp olive oil

4 tofu chops

2 tbsp butter

2 cups chopped beet greens

Directions:

Preheat the oven to 400 F.

In a small saucepan, add the vinegar, salt, black pepper, garlic, and basil. Cook over low heat until the mixture is syrupy. Turn the heat off.

Heat the olive oil in a medium : safe ovenskillet and sear the tofu on both sides until brown, 6 to 8 minutes. Brush the vinegar glaze on both sides of the tofu, add the thyme sprigs, and bake in the oven for 8 minutes or until the tofu cooks within.

Meanwhile, melt the butter in another skillet and sauté the beetroot greens until softened. Season with salt and black pepper, 3 to 5 minutes.

Remove the tofu when ready and serve with the buttered beetroot greens.

Nutrition:

Calories:286, Total Fat:27g, Saturated Fat:15g, Total Carbs:5g, Dietary Fiber:0g, Sugar:1g, Protein:9g, Sodium:87mg

# 56. BBQ Baked Tempeh Chops

Preparation Time: 10minutes

Cooking Time: 58minutes

Servings: 4

Ingredients:

½ cup grated flaxseed meal

1 tsp dried thyme

1 tsp paprika

Salt and ground black pepper to taste

¼ tsp chili powder

1 ½ tsp garlic powder

1 tbsp dried parsley

1/2 tsp onion powder

1/8 tsp basil

4 tempeh chops

1 tbsp melted butter

½ cup unsweetened BBQ sauce

Directions:

Preheat the oven to 400 F and grease a baking sheet with cooking spray. Set aside.

In a medium bowl, mix the flaxseed meal, thyme, paprika, salt, black pepper, chili powder, garlic powder, parsley, onion powder, and basil.

Rub the tempeh chops with the mixture on all sides.

Melt the butter in a medium skillet and sear the tempeh on both sides, 8 minutes. Transfer to the baking sheet, baste with BBQ sauce and bake in the oven for 50 minutes or until the internal temperature reaches 150 F.

Remove the tempeh, allow resting for 10 minutes, slice, and serve with buttered parsnips.

Nutrition:

Calories:376, Total Fat:36.2g, Saturated Fat:23.2g, Total Carbs:3g, Dietary Fiber:0g, Sugar:2g, Protein:11g, Sodium:925mg

## 57. Chipotle-Coffee Tempeh Chops

Preparation Time: 5minutes

Cooking Time: 13minutes

Servings: 4

Ingredients:

1 tbsp finely ground coffee

½ tsp chipotle powder

½ tsp garlic powder

½ tsp cinnamon powder

½ tsp cumin powder

Salt and black pepper to taste

1 ½ tsp swerve brown sugar

4 tempeh chops

2 tbsp lard

Directions:

In a medium bowl, mix the coffee, chipotle powder, garlic, cinnamon, cumin, salt, black pepper, and swerve sugar. Pat the meat dry and rub the spice mixture all over. Cover with plastic wraps and marinate in the fridge overnight.

Preheat the oven to 350 F and remove the tempeh, unwrap, and allow sitting for 30 minutes before cooking.

Melt the lard in a medium safe oven skillet and sear the meat on both sides for 2 to 3 minutes. Transfer to the skillet with meat to the oven and bake for 10 minutes or until the meat's temperature reaches 145 F.

Remove the meat from the oven, place on a cutting board, and allow cooling for 5 minutes.

Slice and serve with buttered snap peas.

Nutrition:

Calories163:, Total Fat:9.9g, Saturated Fat:5.6g, Total Carbs:7g, Dietary Fiber:2g, Sugar:4g, Protein:13g, Sodium:471mg

## 58. Mushroom Crackling with Coconut Creamed Kale

Preparation Time: 20minutes

Cooking Time: 20minutes

Servings: 4

Ingredients:

2 lb mushroom

Salt and black pepper to taste

2 cups water

1 tbsp coconut oil

1 medium white onion finely chopped

6 cloves garlic finely chopped

¼ cup ginger thinly sliced

4 long red chilies, halved

1 cup coconut milk

1 cup coconut cream

2 cups chopped kale

Directions:

Pat the mushroom dry with paper towel, cut into bite-size pieces, and season with salt and black pepper. Place in a bowl and marinate in the refrigerator for 20 to 30 minutes.

Pour the water in a medium pot, add the mushroom and bring to a boil over medium heat until the meat is tender, 10 to 15 minutes. Drain the liquid through a colander and transfer the mushroom to a large skillet.

Fry the mushroom over medium heat : in its fatfor about 16 minutes. The goal is to fry the meat until the skin browns and crackles. Turn a few times to prevent the meat from burning. Spoon the meat onto a plate and discard the fat.

Heat the coconut oil in the same skillet and sauté the onion, garlic, ginger, and red chilies until softened, 5 minutes.

Pour in the coconut milk and cream and allow cooking over low heat for 1 minute. Add the kale and cook until wilted, while stirring occasionally. Season with salt and black pepper; stir in the mushroom until well combined. Cook for 1 to 2 minutes and turn the heat off.

Dish the food into serving plates and serve warm with low carb bread.

Nutrition:

Calories:232, Total Fat:14.3g, Saturated Fat:5.4g, Total Carbs:12g, Dietary Fiber:4g, Sugar:4g, Protein:20g, Sodium:719mg

# 59. Tofu with Morels

Preparation Time: 5minutes

Cooking Time: 10minutes

Servings: 4

Ingredients:

2 tbsp olive oil

1 ½ lb tofu, cut into 8 slices

Salt and black pepper to taste

16 fresh morels, rinsed

4 large green onions, chopped

½ cup red wine

¾ cup vegetable broth

2 tbsp unsalted butter

Directions:

Heat the olive oil in a medium pot, season the tofu medallions with salt and black pepper, and sear in the oil on both sides until brown, 2 to 3 minutes. Transfer to a plate and set aside.

Add the morels and green onions to the pot; cook until softened, 2 minutes and mix in the red wine and vegetable broth.

Place the tofu in the sauce and simmer for 3 to 5 minutes or until the meat cooks.

Swirl in the butter, adjust the taste with salt and black pepper, and dish the food.

Serve immediately with creamy mashed turnips.

Nutrition:

Calories:239, Total Fat:14.7g, Saturated Fat:8.1g, Total Carbs:14g, Dietary Fiber:1g, Sugar:7g, Protein:13g, Sodium:530mg

# 60. Seitan Mozzarella

Preparation Time: 15minutes

Cooking Time: 15minutes

Servings: 4

Ingredients:

4 seitan chops

Salt and black pepper to taste

1 cup golden flaxseed meal

1 large egg, beaten

1 cup unsweetened tomato sauce

1 cup shredded mozzarella cheese

Directions:

Preheat the oven to 400 F and grease a baking sheet with cooking spray. Set aside.

Season the seitan with salt and black pepper, and pour the flaxseed meal onto a plate.

Coat the meat in the egg, then in the flaxseed meal and place on the baking sheet.

Pour the tomato sauce on the meat and sprinkle with the mozzarella cheese. Bake in the oven 10 to 15 minutes or until the cheese melts and seitan cooks through.

Remove from the oven and serve immediately with lettuce salad.

Nutrition:

Calories:492, Total Fat:26.8g, Saturated Fat:12.6g, Total Carbs:14g, Dietary Fiber:4g, Sugar:8g, Protein:50g, Sodium:1668mg

# 61. Vegan Bacon Florentine Pizza

Preparation Time: 10minutes

Cooking Time: 25minutes

Servings: 2

Ingredients:

For the pizza crust:

6 eggs

1 cup shredded provolone cheese

1 tsp Italian seasoning

For the topping:

6 vegan bacon slices

2/3 cup tomato sauce

2 cups chopped kale, wilted

½ cup grated mozzarella cheese

1 : 7 ozcan sliced mushrooms, drained

4 eggs

Olive oil for drizzling

Directions:

For the pizza crust:

Preheat the oven to 400 F and line a pizza-baking pan with parchment paper. Set aside.

Crack the eggs into a medium bowl; whisk in the provolone cheese, and Italian seasoning. Spread the mixture on a pizza-baking pan and bake until golden, 15 minutes. Remove from the oven and allow cooling for 2 minutes.

For the topping:

Increase the oven's temperature to 450 F.

Fry the vegan bacon in a small skillet over medium heat until brown and crispy, 5 minutes. Transfer to a plate pand set aside.

Spread the tomato sauce on the crust, top with the kale, mozzarella, and mushrooms. Bake in the oven for 8 minutes.

Crack the eggs on top, top with the bacon, and continue baking until the eggs set, 2 to 3 minutes.

Remove the pizza, slice, and serve.

Nutrition:

Calories:89, Total Fat:6.4g, Saturated Fat:1.5g, Total Carbs:2g, Dietary Fiber:0g, Sugar:1g, Protein:6g, Sodium:406mg

## 62. Tofu and Walnut Stir-Fry

Preparation Time: 5minutes

Cooking Time: 16minutes

Servings: 4

Ingredients:

2 tbsp coconut oil

1 ½ lb tofu, cut into strips

Salt and black pepper to taste

1 green bell pepper, deseeded and diced

1 small red onion, diced

1/3 cup walnuts

1 tbsp freshly grated ginger

3 garlic cloves, minced

1 tsp sesame oil

1 habanero pepper, minced

2 tbsp tamari sauce

Directions:

Heat the coconut oil in a medium wok over medium heat, season the tofu with salt and black pepper, and cook until no longer pink, 10 minutes.

Shift to one side of the wok and add the bell pepper, onion, walnuts, ginger, garlic, sesame oil, and habanero pepper. Sauté until fragrant, and the onion softened, 5 minutes.

Mix with the tofu and season with the tamari sauce. Stir-fry until well combined and allow cooking for 1 minute.

Spoon the stir-fry into serving plates and serve warm with cauliflower rice.

Nutrition:

Calories:417, Total Fat:36.4g, Saturated Fat:15.9g, Total Carbs:4g, Dietary Fiber:0g, Sugar:1g, Protein:20g, Sodium:525mg

## 63. Herby Lemon Greek Tenderloin

Preparation Time: 1hour, 10minutes

Cooking Time: 50minutes

Servings: 4

Ingredients:

¼ cup olive oil

2 lemon, juiced

2 tbsp Greek seasoning

2 tbsp red wine vinegar

Salt and black pepper to taste

1 ½ lb seitan tenderloin

2 tbsp lard

Directions:

Preheat the oven to 425 F and grease a baking dish with cooking spray. Set aside.

In a medium bowl, combine the olive oil, lemon juice, Greek seasoning, vinegar, salt, and black pepper.

Place the seitan on a clean flat surface, cut a few incisions on the seitan, and brush the marinade all over. Cover in plastic wrap and marinate in the refrigerator for 1 hour.

Melt the lard in a large skillet over medium heat, remove and unwrap the seitan, and sear the meat until brown on the outside.

Place in the baking sheet, brush with any reserved marinade, and bake for 40 to 50 minutes.

Take out the meat, slice, and serve on a bed of spicy buttered spinach.

Nutrition:

Calories:326, Total Fat:24.9g, Saturated Fat:12.9g, Total Carbs:6g, Dietary Fiber:1g, Sugar:4g, Protein:20g, Sodium:568mg

## 64. Herbed Lemon Garlic Tempeh

Preparation Time: 15minutes

Cooking Time: 15minutes

Servings: 4

Ingredients

4 large, tempeh steaks

Salt to taste

2 tsp lemon pepper seasoning

3 tbsp olive oil

3 tbsp butter

1 cup vegetable stock

6 garlic cloves, minced

8 oz white button mushrooms, chopped

2 tbsp freshly chopped parsley

1 lemon, thinly sliced

Directions:

Pat the tempeh dry with a paper towel and season with salt and lemon pepper seasoning.

Heat 2 tablespoons each of the olive oil and butter in a large skillet over medium heat and cook the tempeh on both sides until brown and cooked through, 10 minutes. Transfer the meat to a plate and set aside.

Add the remaining olive oil and butter to the skillet, pour in half of the vegetable stock  to deglaze the bottom of the pan, add the garlic and mushrooms, and cook until softened, 5 minutes.

Return the tempeh to the skillet, add the lemon slices, and cook while basting the tempeh with the sauce until the liquid reduces by two-thirds.

Spoon the tempeh with sauce into serving plates, garnish with parsley, and serve with steamed green beans.

Nutrition:

Calories:253, Total Fat:18.8g, Saturated Fat:7.8g, Total Carbs:9g, Dietary Fiber:2g, Sugar:2g, Protein:14g, Sodium:583mg

# 65. Red Wine Braised Mushroom

Preparation Time: 15minutes

Cooking Time: 2hours, 4minutes

Servings: 4

Ingredients:

3 tbsp olive oil

Salt and ground black pepper to taste

3 lb mushroom

3 celery stalks, chopped

5 garlic cloves, minced

1 ½ cups crushed tomatoes

½ cup red wine

¼ tsp red chili flakes

¼ cup freshly chopped parsley

Directions:

Preheat the oven to 300 F.

Heat the olive oil in a large Dutch oven, season the mushrooms with salt and black pepper, and brown in the oil on all sides, 3 to 4 minutes. Transfer to a plate and set aside.

Add the celery and garlic to the oil and sauté until softened, 3 minutes.

Return the mushroom to the pot and top with the tomatoes, red wine, and red chili flakes. Cover the lid and put the pot in the oven. Cook for 1 ½ to 2 hours, turning the meat every 30 minutes.

In the last 15 minutes, open the lid of the pot and increase the oven's temperature to 450 F.

Take out the pot, stir in the parsley, adjust the taste with salt and black pepper, and serve the meat with sauce on a bed of creamy mashed cauliflower.

Nutrition:

Calories:438, Total Fat:32g, Saturated Fat:18g, Total Carbs:10g, Dietary Fiber:2g, Sugar:5g, Protein:30g, Sodium:771mg

# 66. Mushroom Tofu Meatballs with Coconut Parsnip Mash

Preparation Time: 15minutes

Cooking Time: 47minutes

Servings: 4

Ingredients:

For the meatballs and sauce:

1 ½ lb ground tofu

2 garlic cloves, minced

2 small red onions, chopped

1 cup cremini mushrooms, finely chopped

1 tsp dried basil

Salt and ground black pepper to taste

½ cup grated Soy cheese

½ almond milk

1 ½ + 1 tbsp olive oil

2 cups unsweetened tomato sauce

4 to 6 fresh basil leaves to garnish

For the coconut parsnip mash:

1 lb parsnips, chopped

1 cup water

Salt and ground black pepper to taste

2 tbsp butter

½ cup coconut cream

¼ cup grated Soy cheese

Directions:

For the meatballs and sauce

Preheat the oven to 350 F and line a baking tray with parchment paper.

In a bowl, add the tofu, half of the garlic, half of the onion, mushrooms, basil, salt, and black pepper; mix with your hands until evenly combined. Mold bite-size balls out of the mixture.

Pour the Soy cheese and almond milk each in two separate bowls.

Dip each ball in the almond milk and then in the Soy cheese. Place on the baking sheet and bake in the oven for 10 minutes or until cooked.

Heat 1 ½ tbsp of olive oil in a medium pot, remove the meatballs from the oven, and fry in the oil until golden brown on all sides. Transfer to a paper towel-lined plate and set aside.

Heat the remaining oil in a saucepan and sauté the remaining onion and garlic; sauté until fragrant and soft.

Pour in the tomato sauce and cook for 20 minutes or until a stew forms.

Add the meatballs, spoon some sauce to cover, and simmer for 5 to 7 minutes.

For the parsnip mash:

In a medium pot, add the parsnips, water, and a little salt. Bring to a boil for 10 minutes or until the parsnips soften. Drain through a colander and pour into a medium bowl.

Add the butter, salt, and black pepper; mash into a puree using a potato mash.

Stir in the coconut cream and Soy cheese until evenly combined.

Spoon the mashed parsnip into serving bowls, top with some meatballs and sauce, and garnish with the basil leaves. Serve warm.

Nutrition:

Calories:556, Total Fat:44g, Saturated Fat:26g, Total Carbs:11g, Dietary Fiber:2g, Sugar:7g, Protein:31g, Sodium:1235mg

## 67. Tofu Meatballs with Creamy Cauli Mash

Preparation Time: 15minutes

Cooking Time: 47minutes

Servings: 4

Ingredients:

For the tofu balls and sauce:

1 lb silken tofu, pressed and cubed

2 garlic cloves, minced

2 small red onions, chopped

1 cup white button mushrooms, chopped

1 tsp dried basil

Salt and black pepper to taste

1 small red bell pepper, deseeded and chopped

½ cup golden flaxseed meal

½ almond milk

1 ½ + 1 tbsp. olive oil

2 cups tomato sauce

4 to 6 fresh basil leaves to garnish

For the cauliflower mash:

1 lb cauliflower, cut into florets

1 cup water, for steaming

Salt and black pepper to taste

2 tbsp butter

½ cup heavy cream

¼ cup grated Soy cheese

Directions:

For the tofu balls and sauce:

Preheat the oven to 350 F and line a baking tray with parchment paper.

In a bowl, add the silken tofu, half of the garlic, half of the onion, mushrooms, basil, salt, and black pepper; mix with your hands until evenly combined. Pour the mixture into a bowl and mold bite-size balls out of the mixture.

Place the flaxseed meal and almond milk each in a shallow dish.

Dip each ball in the almond milk and then in the flaxseed meal. Place on the baking sheet and bake in the oven for 10 minutes or until properly compacted.

Heat 1 ½ tbsp of olive oil in a medium pot, remove the tofu balls from the oven, and fry in the oil until golden brown on all sides and compacted. Remove onto a paper towel-lined plate and set aside.

Heat the remaining oil in a saucepan and sauté the onion, garlic, and bell pepper into the oil and sauté until fragrant and soft. Pour in the tomato sauce and cook 20 minutes or until s stew forms. Add the tofu balls, spoon some sauce to cover, and simmer for 5 to 7 minutes.

For the cauliflower mash:

In a medium pot, add the cauliflower, water, and a little salt. Bring to a boil for 10 minutes or until the vegetable softens. Drain through a colander and pour into a medium bowl.

Add the butter, salt, and black pepper; mash into a puree using a potato mash.

Stir in the heavy cream and Soy cheese until evenly combined.

Spoon the cauli mash into serving bowls, top with some tofu balls and sauce, and garnish with the basil leaves. Serve warm.

Nutrition:

Calories:131, Total Fat:10.5g, Saturated Fat:4.3g, Total Carbs:3g, Dietary Fiber:1g, Sugar:1g, Protein:7g, Sodium:375mg

## 68. Tofu Nuggets with Cilantro Dip

Preparation Time: 10minutes

Cooking Time: 15minutes

Servings: 4

Ingredients:

For the tofu nuggets:

1 ½ cups olive oil for frying

2 : 14 ozblocks extra firm tofu, pressed and cut into bite-size cubes

1 egg, lightly beaten

1 cup golden flaxseed meal, seasoned

For the cilantro dip:

1 ripe avocado, halved, pitted, and frozen

½ tbsp. chopped cilantro

Salt and black pepper

½ tbsp. olive oil

1 lime, ½ juiced and ½ cut into wedges for serving

Directions:

For the tofu nuggets:

Heat the olive oil in a large deep skillet.

Meanwhile, coat the tofu cubes in the egg and then adequately in the flaxseed meal. Fry in the hot oil in batches until golden brown on all sides. Transfer to a paper towel-lined plate.

For the cilantro dip.

Place the avocado, cilantro, salt, black pepper, and lime juice in a blender; puree until very smooth.

Spoon the dip into a serving bowl, plate with the tofu nuggets, garnish with the lime wedges, and serve immediately.

Nutrition:

Calories:446, Total Fat:26.3g, Saturated Fat:12.9g, Total Carbs:13g, Dietary Fiber:3g, Sugar:7g, Protein:42g, Sodium:1011mg

# 69. Zucchini- Cranberry Cake Squares

Preparation Time: 17minutes

Cooking Time: 15minutes

Servings: 6

Ingredients:

1 ¼ cup chopped zucchinis

2 tbsp olive oil

½ cup dried cranberries

1 lemon, zested

3 eggs

1 ½ cups almond flour

½ tsp baking powder

1 tsp cinnamon powder

A pinch salt

Directions:

Preheat the oven to 350 F and line a square cake tin with parchment paper.

Pour the zucchinis into a colander, sprinkle with salt, and allow sitting for 5 minutes. After, squeeze out as much liquid from the vegetable and transfer to a large mixing bowl.

Add the olive oil, cranberries, lemon zest, and eggs until evenly combined.

Sift the flour, baking powder, and cinnamon powder into the mixture and fold with the salt.

Pour the mixture into the cake tin and bake in the oven for 30 minutes or until the cake turns golden and a toothpick inserted into the cake comes out clean.

Remove; allow cooling in the tin for 10 minutes and transfer the cake to a wire rack to cool completely.

Cut into squares and serve the kids for snack.

Nutrition:

Calories:255, Total Fat:14.6g, Saturated Fat:6.7g, Total Carbs:10g, Dietary Fiber:2g, Sugar:3g, Protein:23g, Sodium:684mg

# 70. Strawberry Faux Oats

Preparation Time: 10minutes

Cooking Time: 10minutes

Serving size 2

Ingredients:

2 tbsp coconut flour

2 tbsp golden flaxseed meal

2 tbsp chia seeds

2 tbsp heavy cream

½ cup almond milk

3 tbsp sugar-free maple syrup

1 tsp vanilla extract

1 cup frozen strawberries, halved

¼ cup desiccated coconut

Directions:

Combine the coconut flour, flaxseed meal, and chia seeds in a small saucepan. Stir in the heavy cream, almond milk, maple syrup, and vanilla extract.

Place the pan over medium heat, whisk the Ingredients until thick and warmed through, 10 minutes.

Pour the mixture into two serving bowls and top with the strawberries and desiccated coconut. Drizzle with some more maple syrup for more sweetness and serve warm.

Nutrition:

Calories:122, Total Fat:9.9g, Saturated Fat:1.3g, Total Carbs:3g, Dietary Fiber:1g, Sugar:1g, Protein:6g, Sodium:201mg

## 71. Creamy Paprika Seitan

Preparation Time: 10minutes

Cooking Time: 12minutes

Servings: 4

Ingredients:

1 lb seitan, cut into 1-inch cubes

4 tsp smoked paprika

Salt and black pepper to taste

1 tsp almond flour

1 tbsp butter

3/4 cup coconut cream

Directions:

Pat dry the seitan pieces with a paper towel and season with paprika, salt, black pepper, and sprinkle with the almond flour.

Melt the butter in a large skillet and sauté the seitan until lightly browned, 4 to 5 minutes.

Pour in the coconut cream; allow boiling while stirring to loosen the browned bits from the pan. Cook without covering until the sauce slightly thickens, 5 to 7 minutes. Adjust the taste with salt and black pepper.

Dish the food over a bed of cauliflower rice. Serve immediately.

Nutrition:

Calories:248, Total Fat:22.7g, Saturated Fat:1g, Total Carbs:5g, Dietary Fiber:3g, Sugar:1g, Protein:9g, Sodium:227mg

## 72. Tempeh Chops with Garlic-Raspberry Sauce

Preparation Time: 17minutes

Cooking Time: 10minutes

Servings: 4

Ingredients:

2 cups fresh raspberries

¼ cup water

1 tsp mushroom granules

½ cup almond flour

2 large eggs, lightly beaten

2/3 cup grated Soy cheese

1 lb tempeh, cut into ½ -inch medallions

Salt and ground black pepper to taste

6 tbsp butter, divided

1 tsp minced garlic

Sliced fresh raspberries, optional

Directions:

Into a blender, add the raspberries, water, and mushroom granules and process until smooth. Set aside.

In two separate bowls, pour the almond flour and Soy cheese. Season the tempeh with salt and black pepper. Coat the tempeh in the almond flour, then in the eggs, and then generously in the Soy cheese.

Melt 2 tablespoons of the butter in a large skillet over medium heat and fry the tempeh for 2 to 3 minutes on each side or until the cheese melts and the tempeh cooks within. Transfer to a plate, cover and keep warm.

In the same skillet, melt the remaining butter and sauté the garlic for 1 minute. Stir in the raspberry mixture and cook for 2 to 3 minutes.

Dish the tempeh into serving plates and spoon the sauce on top. Garnish with the raspberries and serve immediately with baby spinach.

Nutrition:

Calories:452, Total Fat:38.2g, Saturated Fat:19.5g, Total Carbs:6g, Dietary Fiber:1g, Sugar:2g, Protein:23g, Sodium:746mg

# 73. Mediterranean Tofu and Cauliflower Rice

Preparation Time: 10minutes

Cooking Time: 11minutes

Servings: 4

Ingredients:

2 tbsp olive oil

1 ½ lb tofu, cut into 1-inch cubes

Salt and ground black pepper to taste

½ tsp cumin powder

2 cups cauliflower rice

½ cup water

1 cup loosely packed fresh baby spinach

1 cup grape tomatoes, halved

3/4 cup crumbled feta cheese

Directions:

Heat the olive oil in a large skillet, season the tofu with salt, black pepper, and cumin, and sear on both sides for 3 to 5 minutes or until the meat browns.

Stir in the cauliflower rice, season with more salt and black pepper, and pour in the water. Cook for 5 minutes or until the cauliflower softens.

Mix in the spinach to wilt, 1 minute and add the tomatoes.

Spoon the dish into serving bowls, sprinkle with the feta cheese, and serve with hot sauce.

Nutrition:

Calories:79, Total Fat:6.2g, Saturated Fat:3.7g, Total Carbs:5g, Dietary Fiber:2g, Sugar:3g, Protein:2g, Sodium:54mg

## 74. Mushroom Masala

Prep Time 10minutes

Cooking Time 18minutes

Serving size 4

Ingredients:

1 ½ lb mushroom, cut into bite-size pieces

2 tbsp ghee

1 tbsp freshly grated ginger

2 tbsp freshly pureed garlic

6 medium red onions, thinly sliced

1 cup crushed tomatoes

2 tbsp Greek sugar free coconut yogurt

½ tsp chili powder

2 tbsp garam masala

Salt and ground black pepper to taste

1 bunch coriander, chopped

2 green chilies, sliced

Directions:

Bring a large pot of water to the boil and blanch the mushroom for 3 minutes. Drain and set aside.

Melt the ghee in a large skillet and sauté the ginger, garlic, and onions until the onions caramelize, 5 minutes.

Mix in the tomatoes, sugar free coconut yogurt, and mushroom. Season with the chili powder, garam masala, salt, and black pepper. Stir well and cook for about 10 minutes.

Adjust the taste with salt and black pepper and stir in the coriander and green chilies.

Serve the masala with cauliflower rice.

Nutrition:

Calories:408, Total Fat:39.5g, Saturated Fat:24.4g, Total Carbs:8g, Dietary Fiber:1g, Sugar:2g, Protein:8g, Sodium:543mg

## 75. Tempeh Taco Cups

Preparation Time: 10minutes

Cooking Time: 21minutes

Servings: 4

Ingredients:

4 low carb tortilla wraps

2 tsp melted butter

1 tbsp olive oil

1 small yellow onion, finely chopped

½ cup tempeh, crumbled

1 tsp smoked paprika

½ tsp cumin powder

Salt and black pepper to taste

1 small iceberg lettuce, 8 firm leaves extracted

1 medium red bell pepper, deseeded and chopped

1 ripe avocado, halved and pitted

1 small lemon, juiced

¼ cup sour cream

Directions:

Preheat the oven to 400 F.

Divide each tortilla wrap into two, lay on a chopping board, and brush with butter. Line 8 muffin tins with the tortilla and bake in the oven for 8 to 9 minutes or until the edges crisp and lightly golden. Remove from the oven and set aside to cool.

Heat the olive oil in a skillet and sauté the onion for 3 minutes. Crumble the tempeh into the pan and cook for 8 minutes or until deep brown. Stir in the paprika, cumin, salt, black pepper and cook for 1 minute.

To assemble, fit the lettuce leaves into the tortilla cups, share the tempeh mixture on top, top with the bell pepper, avocado, and drizzle with the lemon juice. Add the sour cream and serve immediately.

Nutrition:

Calories:105, Total Fat:11.6g, Saturated Fat:7.3g, Total Carbs:1g, Dietary Fiber:0g, Sugar:0g, Protein:0g, Sodium:238mg

## 76. Cheese Quesadillas with Fruit Salad

Preparation Time: 5minutes

Cooking Time: 2minutes

Serving size 2

Ingredients:

For the quesadillas:

2 large low carb tortillas

1 cup grated cheddar cheese

2 small green onions, chopped

For the fruit salad:

1 cup mixed berries

½ tsp cinnamon powder

½ lemon, juiced

1 cup Greek sugar free coconut yogurt

Sugar-free maple syrup to taste

Directions:

Divide the tortillas into two, top half each with the cheddar cheese and spring onion, and cover with the halves.

Place in a large non- stick skillet and heat until golden and the cheese melted. Remove onto a plate, allow cooling, and cut into four wedges.

For the salad, combine the berries, cinnamon powder, lemon juice, Greek sugar free coconut yogurt, and maple syrup in a bowl. Divide into two bowls and serve with the quesadillas.

Nutrition:

Calories:442, Total Fat:29.4g, Saturated Fat:11.3g, Total Carbs:8g, Dietary Fiber:1g, Sugar:1g, Protein:39g, Sodium:814mg

# 77. Cauliflower and Halloumi Packets

Preparation Time: 10minutes

Cooking Time: 15minutes

Servings: 4

Ingredients:

2 heads cauliflower, chopped roughly

¼ cup vegetable broth

1 lemon, juiced

2 tbsp sugar-free maple syrup

1 red bell pepper, deseeded and chopped

1 orange bell pepper, deseeded and chopped

¼ cup cubed halloumi

Olive oil to drizzle

Directions:

Place a baking tray in the oven and preheat the oven to 350 F.

Place the cauliflower in a food processor and pulse a few times until a coarse consistency is achieved but not riced to make the couscous.

Pour the couscous and vegetable stock into a medium pot; cook over medium heat until slightly softened, 2 to 3 minutes. Drain afterwards using a sieve and set aside.

In a small bowl, whisk the lemon juice and maple syrup, and set aside.

Cut out two 2 x 15 inches parchment papers onto a flat surface spoon the couscous in the middle of each, top with the bell peppers, halloumi, and drizzle the dressing on top. Add more olive oil as desired.

Wrap the papers into parcels and place on the baking tray; cook for 10 to 15 minutes.

When ready, remove and carefully open the pouches to allow the steam escape.

Serve warm to the kids.

Nutrition:

Calories314:, Total Fat:30.6g, Saturated Fat:12.3g, Total Carbs:8g, Dietary Fiber:2g, Sugar:4g, Protein:5g, Sodium:37mg

## 78. Tofu Cabbage Stew

Preparation Time: 30minutes

Cooking Time: 15minutes | Serving: 4

Ingredients:

5 oz. butter

2 ½ cups baby bok choy, quartered lengthwise

2 cups water packed extra firm tofu

1 tsp salt

¼ tsp black pepper

1 tsp garlic powder

1 tsp onion powder

1 tbsp plain vinegar

2 garlic cloves, minced

1 tsp chili flakes

1 tbsp fresh ginger, grated

3 green onions, sliced

1 tbsp sesame oil

Wasabi mayonnaise

1 cup vegan mayonnaise

½ - 1 tbsp wasabi paste

Directions:

Place the tofu in between two paper towels and allow to drain liquid for 30 minutes. After, cut into 1-inch cubes and set aside.

Melt half of the butter in a wok over medium heat, add the bok choy, and stir-fry until softened.

Season with the salt, black pepper, garlic powder, onion powder, and plain vinegar. Sauté for 2 minutes to combine the flavors and then, spoon the bok choy into a bowl. Set aside.

Melt the remaining butter in the wok, add and sauté the garlic, chili flakes, and ginger until fragrant.

Put the tofu in the wok and cook until browned on all sides. Add the green onions and bok Choy, heat for 2 minutes and add the sesame oil.

Combine the mayonnaise and wasabi in a small bowl and stir the mixture in small portions into the wok until tasty as desired. Cook for 1 minute and dish the stir-fry.

Serve with steamed cauli rice.

Nutrition:

Calories:232, Total Fat:14.3g, Saturated Fat:5.4g, Total Carbs:12g, Dietary Fiber:4g, Sugar:4g, Protein:20g, Sodium:719mg

## 79. Curried Tofu with Buttery Cabbage

Preparation Time: 35minutes

Cooking Time: 20minutes

Servings: 4

Ingredients:

2 cups water packed extra firm tofu

1 tbsp + 3 ½ tbsp coconut oil

½ cup unsweetened shredded coconut

1 tsp yellow curry powder

1 tsp salt

½ tsp onion powder

2 cups Napa cabbage

4 oz. butter

Salt and black pepper

Lemon wedges for serving

Directions:

Place the tofu in between two paper towels to drain liquid for 30 minutes. After, cut into bite-size cubes and drizzle 1 tablespoon of coconut oil on the tofu.

In a bowl, mix the shredded coconut, yellow curry powder, salt, and onion powder. Then, toss the tofu cubes in the spice mixture.

Heat the remaining coconut oil in a non-stick skillet and fry the coated tofu until golden brown on all sides. Transfer to a plate to keep warm.

In another skillet, melt half of the butter, add, and sauté the cabbage until slightly caramelized. Then, season with salt and black pepper.

Dish the cabbage into serving plates with the tofu and lemon wedges.

Melt the remaining butter in the skillet and drizzle over the cabbage and tofu.

Serve immediately.

Nutrition:

Calories:673, Total Fat:58.8g, Saturated Fat:36.3g, Total Carbs:16g, Dietary Fiber:7g, Sugar:2g, Protein:26g, Sodium:760mg

## 80. Tofu Radish Bowls

Preparation Time: 15minutes

Cooking Time: 20minutes

Servings: 4

Ingredients:

1 tbsp + 1 tbsp olive oil

1 : 14 ozblock extra firm tofu, pressed and cubed

1 ½ cup shredded radishes

½ cup chopped white onions

2 yellow bell peppers, deseeded and chopped

Salt and black pepper to taste

¼ cup chopped baby bella mushrooms

4 eggs

1/3 cup tomato salsa

A handful chopped parsley

1 ripe avocado, pitted and chopped

Directions:

Heat 1 tablespoon of olive oil in a skillet over medium heat and add the tofu, radishes, onions, and bell peppers. Season with salt and black pepper; cook for 4 minutes on each side or until the tofu is slightly golden.

Pour in the mushrooms, continue cooking until the vegetable crisp and turn golden brown. Divide into four bowls.

Heat the remaining olive oil in the skillet, crack an egg each into the pan, and cook until the white sets, but the yolk quite runny.

Transfer to the top of one tofu-radish hash bowl and make the remaining eggs.

Top the bowls with the tomato salsa, parsley, and avocado. Serve immediately.

Nutrition:

Calories:239, Total Fat:14.7g, Saturated Fat:8.1g, Total Carbs:14g, Dietary Fiber:1g, Sugar:7g, Protein:13g, Sodium:530mg

# 81. Cheesy Broccoli Nachos with Salsa

Preparation Time: 10minutes

Cooking Time: 20minutes

Servings: 4

Ingredients:

For the cheesy broccoli nachos:

2 heads medium broccoli, trimmed and chopped

3 tbsp coconut flour

1 tsp smoked paprika

½ tsp coriander powder

1 tsp cumin powder

½ tsp garlic powder

2 eggs, beaten

¼ cup grated Monterey jack cheese

For the salsa:

4 plum tomatoes, finely chopped

½ lime, juiced

4 sprigs cilantro, chopped

1 avocado, halved, pitted, and chopped

Directions:

Preheat the oven to 350 F.

Pour the broccoli into a food processor and blend into a rice-like consistency. Heat a large skillet over low heat, pour in the broccoli, and dry-fry for 10 minutes or until most of the moisture has evaporated. Transfer to a mixing bowl to cool.

Line two baking sheets with parchment papers and set aside.

Onto the broccoli, add the coconut flour, smoked paprika, coriander powder, cumin powder, garlic powder, and eggs. Mix and use your hands to form into a ball.

Divide into halves, place each half on each baking sheet, and press down into a rough circle. Bake in the oven for 5 to 10 minutes or until golden on both sides.

Take out of the oven, cut into triangles immediately, and sprinkle with the cheese. Allow cooling while you make the salsa.

In a bowl, combine the tomatoes, lime, cilantro, and avocado.

Serve the nachos with the salsa

Nutrition:

Calories:89, Total Fat:6.4g, Saturated Fat:1.5g, Total Carbs:2g, Dietary Fiber:0g, Sugar:1g, Protein:6g, Sodium:406mg

## 82. Cheesy Cauliflower Casserole

Preparation Time: 14minutes

Cooking Time: 20minutes

Servings: 4

Ingredients:

2 oz. butter

1 white onion, finely chopped

½ cup celery stalks, finely chopped

1 green bell pepper, seeded and finely chopped

Salt and black pepper

1 small head cauliflower, chopped

1 cup vegan mayonnaise

4 oz. freshly shredded parmesan cheese

1 tsp red chili flakes

Directions:

Preheat the oven to 400 F and grease a baking dish with cooking spray.

Season the onion, celery, and bell pepper with salt and black pepper.

In a bowl, mix the cauliflower, mayonnaise, parmesan cheese, and red chili flakes.

Pour the mixture into the baking dish, add the season vegetables, and mix to be evenly distributed.

Bake in the oven until golden brown, about 20 minutes.

Remove the cauli bake and serve warm with baby spinach.

Nutrition:

Calories:417, Total Fat:36.4g, Saturated Fat:15.9g, Total Carbs:4g, Dietary Fiber:0g, Sugar:1g, Protein:20g, Sodium:525mg

## 83. Creamy Brussels Sprouts Bowls

Preparation time: 10 minutes

Cooking time: 30 minutes

Servings: 4

Ingredients:

1 tablespoon olive oil

1 pound Brussels sprouts, trimmed and halved

1 cup coconut cream

½ teaspoon chili powder

½ teaspoon garam masala

½ teaspoon garlic powder

A pinch of salt and black pepper

1 tablespoon lime juice

Directions:

In a roasting pan, combine the sprouts with the cream, chili powder and the other ingredients, toss, introduce in the oven at 380 degrees F and bake for 30 minutes.

Divide into bowls and serve for lunch.

Nutrition: calories 219, fat 18.3, fiber 5.7, carbs 14.1, protein 5.4

## 84. Green Beans and Radishes Bake

Preparation time: 10 minutes

Cooking time: 25 minutes

Servings: 4

Ingredients:

2 tablespoons olive oil

1 pound green beans, trimmed and halved

2 cups radishes, sliced

1 cup coconut cream

1 teaspoon sweet paprika

1 cup cashew cheese, shredded

Salt and black pepper to the taste

1 tablespoon chives, chopped

Directions:

In a roasting pan, combine the green beans with the radishes and the other ingredients except the cheese and toss.

Sprinkle the cheese on top, introduce in the oven at 375 degrees F and bake for 25 minutes.

Divide the mix between plates and serve.

Nutrition: calories 130, fat 1, fiber 0.4, carbs 1, protein 0.1

## 85. Avocado and Radish Bowls

Preparation time: 10 minutes

Cooking time: 0 minutes

Servings: 4

Ingredients:

2 cups radishes, halved

2 avocados, peeled, pitted and roughly cubed

2 tablespoons coconut cream

2 tablespoons balsamic vinegar

1 tablespoon green onion, chopped

1 teaspoon chili powder

1 cup baby spinach

Salt and black pepper to the taste

Directions:

1. In a bowl, combine the radishes with the avocados and the other ingredients, toss, divide into smaller bowls and serve for lunch.

Nutrition: calories 340, fat 23, fiber 3, carbs 6, protein 5

## 86. Celery and Radish Soup

Preparation time: 10 minutes

Cooking time: 20 minutes

Servings: 4

Ingredients:

½ pound radishes, cut into quarters

2 celery stalks, chopped

2 tablespoons olive oil

4 scallions, chopped

1 teaspoon fennel seeds, crushed

1 teaspoon coriander, dried

6 cups vegetable stock

Salt and black pepper to the taste

6 garlic cloves, minced

1 tablespoon chives, chopped

Directions:

Heat up a pot with the oil over medium heat, add the celery, scallions and the garlic and sauté for 5 minutes.

Add the radishes and the other ingredients, bring to a boil, cover and simmer for 15 minutes.

Divide into soup bowls and serve.

Nutrition: calories 120, fat 2, fiber 1, carbs 3, protein 10

## 87. Lime Avocado and Cucumber Soup

Preparation time: 5 minutes

Cooking time: 0 minutes

Servings: 4

Ingredients:

2 avocados, pitted, peeled and roughly cubed

2 cucumbers, sliced

4 cups vegetable stock

Salt and black pepper to the taste

¼ teaspoon lemon zest, grated

1 tablespoon white vinegar

1 cup scallions, chopped

1 tablespoon olive oil

¼ cup cilantro, chopped

Directions:

In a blender, combine the avocados with the cucumbers and the other ingredients, pulse well, divide into bowls and serve for lunch.

Nutrition: calories 100, fat 10, fiber 2, carbs 5, protein 8

# 88. Avocado and Kale Soup

Preparation time: 5 minutes

Cooking time: 7 minutes

Servings: 4

Ingredients:

4 cups kale, torn

1 teaspoon turmeric powder

1 avocado, pitted, peeled and sliced

4 cups vegetable stock

Juice of 1 lime

2 garlic cloves, minced

1 tablespoon chives, chopped

Salt and black pepper to the taste

Directions:

In a pot, combine the kale with the avocado and the other ingredients, bring to a simmer, cook over medium heat for 7 minutes, blend using an immersion blender, divide into bowls and serve.

Nutrition: calories 234, fat 12, fiber 4, carbs 7, protein 12

## 89. Spinach and Cucumber Salad

Preparation time: 5 minutes

Cooking time: 0 minutes

Servings: 4

Ingredients:

1 pound cucumber, sliced

2 cups baby spinach

1 tablespoon chili powder

2 tablespoons olive oil

¼ cup cilantro, chopped

2 tablespoons lemon juice

Salt and black pepper to the taste

Directions:

In a large salad bowl, combine the cucumber with the spinach and the other ingredients, toss and serve for lunch.

Nutrition: calories 140, fat 4, fiber 2, carbs 4, protein 5

## 90. Avocado Soup

Preparation time: 10 minutes

Cooking time: 0 minutes

Servings: 4

Ingredients:

2 avocados, pitted, peeled and chopped

4 cups vegetable stock

2 scallions, chopped

Salt and black pepper to the taste

2 tablespoons coconut oil, melted

2/3 cup coconut cream

Directions:

In a blender, combine the avocados with the stock and the other ingredients, pulse well, divide into bowls and serve.

Nutrition: calories 332, fat 23, fiber 4, carbs 6, protein 6

## 91. Avocado, Spinach and Kale Soup

Preparation time: 10 minutes

Cooking time: 0 minutes

Servings: 4

Ingredients:

2 avocados, pitted, peeled and cut in halves

4 cups vegetable stock

2 tablespoons cilantro, chopped

Juice of 1 lime

1 teaspoon rosemary, dried

½ cup spinach leaves

½ cup kale, torn

Salt and black pepper to the taste

Directions:

1. In a blender, combine the avocados with the stock and the other ingredients, pulse well, divide into bowls and serve for lunch.

Nutrition: calories 300, fat 23, fiber 5, carbs 6, protein 7

## 92. Curry Spinach Soup

Preparation time: 10 minutes

Cooking time: 0 minutes

Servings: 4

Ingredients:

1 cup almond milk

1 tablespoon green curry paste

1 pound spinach leaves

1 tablespoon cilantro, chopped

Salt and black pepper to the taste

4 cups veggie stock

1 tablespoon cilantro, chopped

Directions:

In your blender, combine the almond milk with the curry paste and the other ingredients, pulse well, divide into bowls and serve for lunch.

Nutrition: calories 240, fat 4, fiber 2, carbs 6, protein 2

## 93. Arugula and Artichokes Bowls

Preparation time: 5 minutes

Cooking time: 0 minutes

Servings: 4

Ingredients:

2 cups baby arugula

¼ cup walnuts, chopped

1 cup canned artichoke hearts, drained and quartered

1 tablespoon balsamic vinegar

2 tablespoons cilantro, chopped

2 tablespoons olive oil

Salt and black pepper to the taste

1 tablespoon lemon juice

Directions:

In a bowl, combine the artichokes with the arugula, walnuts and the other ingredients, toss, divide into smaller bowls and serve for lunch.

Nutrition: calories 200, fat 2, fiber 1, carbs 5, protein 7

## 94. Minty Arugula Soup

Preparation time: 5 minutes

Cooking time: 10 minutes

Servings: 4

Ingredients:

3 scallions, chopped

1 tablespoon olive oil

½ cup coconut milk

2 cups baby arugula

2 tablespoons mint, chopped

6 cups vegetable stock

2 tablespoons chives, chopped

Salt and black pepper to the taste

Directions:

Heat up a pot with the oil over medium high heat, add the scallions and sauté for 2 minutes.

Add the rest of the ingredients, toss, bring to a simmer and cook over medium heat for 8 minutes more.

Divide the soup into bowls and serve.

Nutrition: calories 200, fat 4, fiber 2, carbs 6, protein 10

## 95. Spinach and Broccoli Soup

Preparation time: 10 minutes

Cooking time: 20 minutes

Servings: 4

Ingredients:

3 shallots, chopped

1 tablespoon olive oil

2 garlic cloves, minced

½ pound broccoli florets

½ pound baby spinach

Salt and black pepper to the taste

4 cups veggie stock

1 teaspoon turmeric powder

1 tablespoon lime juice

Directions:

Heat up a pot with the oil over medium high heat, add the shallots and the garlic and sauté for 5 minutes.

Add the broccoli, spinach and the other ingredients, toss, bring to a simmer and cook over medium heat for 15 minutes.

Ladle into soup bowls and serve.

Nutrition: calories 150, fat 3, fiber 1, carbs 3, protein 7

# 96. Coconut Zucchini Cream

!

Preparation time: 10 minutes

Cooking time: 25 minutes

Servings: 4

Ingredients:

1 pound zucchinis, roughly chopped

2 tablespoons avocado oil

4 scallions, chopped

Salt and black pepper to the taste

6 cups veggie stock

1 teaspoon basil, dried

1 teaspoon cumin, ground

3 garlic cloves, minced

¾ cup coconut cream

1 tablespoon dill, chopped

Directions:

Heat up a pot with the oil over medium high heat, add the scallions and the garlic and sauté for 5 minutes.

Add the rest of the ingredients, stir, bring to a simmer and cook over medium heat for 20 minutes more.

Blend the soup using an immersion blender, ladle into bowls and serve.

Nutrition: calories 160, fat 4, fiber 2, carbs 4, protein 8

## 97. Zucchini and Cauliflower Soup

Preparation time: 10 minutes

Cooking time: 25 minutes

Servings: 4

Ingredients:

4 scallions, chopped

1 teaspoon ginger, grated

2 tablespoons olive oil

1 pound zucchinis, sliced

2 cups cauliflower florets

Salt and black pepper to the taste

6 cups veggie stock

1 garlic clove, minced

1 tablespoon lemon juice

1 cup coconut cream

Directions:

Heat up a pot with the oil over medium heat, add the scallions, ginger and the garlic and sauté for 5 minutes.

Add the rest of the ingredients, bring to a simmer and cook over medium heat for 20 minutes.

Blend everything using an immersion blender, ladle into soup bowls and serve.

Nutrition: calories 154, fat 12, fiber 3, carbs 5, protein 4

## 98. Chard Soup

Preparation time: 10 minutes

Cooking time: 25 minutes

Servings: 4

Ingredients:

1 pound Swiss chard, chopped

½ cup shallots, chopped

1 tablespoon avocado oil

1 teaspoon cumin, ground

1 teaspoon rosemary, dried

1 teaspoon basil, dried

2 garlic cloves, minced

Salt and black pepper to the taste

6 cups vegetable stock

1 tablespoon tomato passata

1 tablespoon cilantro, chopped

Directions:

Heat up a pan with the oil over medium heat, add the shallots and the garlic and sauté for 5 minutes.

Add the Swiss chard and the other ingredients, toss, bring to a simmer and cook over medium heat for 20 minutes more.

Divide the soup into bowls and serve.

Nutrition: calories 232, fat 23, fiber 3, carbs 4, protein 3

## 99. Avocado, Pine Nuts and Chard Salad

Preparation time: 5 minutes

Cooking time: 15 minutes

Servings: 4

Ingredients:

1 pound Swiss chard, roughly chopped

2 tablespoons olive oil

1 avocado, peeled, pitted and roughly cubed

2 spring onions, chopped

¼ cup pine nuts, toasted

1 tablespoon balsamic vinegar

Salt and black pepper to the taste

Directions:

Heat up a pan with the oil over medium heat, add the spring onions, pine nuts and the chard, stir and sauté for 5 minutes.

Add the vinegar and the other ingredients, toss, cook over medium heat for 10 minutes more, divide into bowls and serve for lunch.

Nutrition: calories 120, fat 2, fiber 1, carbs 4, protein 8

## 100. Grapes, Avocado and Spinach Salad

Preparation time: 10 minutes

Cooking time: 0 minutes

Servings: 4

Ingredients:

1 cup green grapes, halved

2 cups baby spinach

1 avocado, pitted, peeled and cubed

Salt and black pepper to the taste

2 tablespoons olive oil

1 tablespoon thyme, chopped

1 tablespoon rosemary, chopped

1 tablespoon lime juice

1 garlic clove, minced

Directions:

In a salad bowl, combine the grapes with the spinach and the other ingredients, toss, and serve for lunch.

Nutrition: calories 190, fat 17.1, fiber 4.6, carbs 10.9, protein 1.7

## 101. Greens and Olives Pan

Preparation time: 10 minutes

Cooking time: 15 minutes

Servings: 4

Ingredients:

4 spring onions, chopped

2 tablespoons olive oil

½ cup green olives, pitted and halved

¼ cup pine nuts, toasted

1 tablespoon balsamic vinegar

2 cups baby spinach

1 cup baby arugula

1 cup asparagus, trimmed, blanched and halved

Salt and black pepper to the taste

Directions:

Heat up a pan with the oil over medium high heat, add the spring onions and the asparagus and sauté for 5 minutes.

Add the olives, spinach and the other ingredients, toss, cook over medium heat for 10 minutes, divide between plates and serve for lunch.

Nutrition: calories 136, fat 13.1, fiber 1.9, carbs 4.4, protein 2.8

## 102. Mushrooms and Chard Soup

Preparation time: 10 minutes

Cooking time: 30 minutes

Servings: 4

Ingredients:

3 cups Swiss chard, chopped

6 cups vegetable stock

1 cup mushrooms, sliced

2 garlic cloves, minced

1 tablespoon olive oil

2 scallions, chopped

2 tablespoons balsamic vinegar

¼ cup basil, chopped

Salt and black pepper to the taste

1 tablespoon cilantro, chopped

Directions:

Heat up a pot with the oil over medium high heat, add the scallions and the garlic and sauté for 5 minutes.

Add the mushrooms and sauté for another 5 minutes.

Add the rest of the ingredients, toss, bring to a simmer and cook over medium heat for 20 minutes more.

Ladle the soup into bowls and serve.

Nutrition: calories 140, fat 4, fiber 2, carbs 4, protein 8

## 103. Tomato, Green Beans and Chard Soup

Preparation time: 10 minutes

Cooking time: 35 minutes

Servings: 4

Ingredients:

2 scallions, chopped

1 cup Swiss chard, chopped

1 tablespoon olive oil

1 red bell pepper, chopped

Salt and black pepper to the taste

1 cup tomatoes, cubed

1 cup green beans, chopped

6 cups vegetable stock

2 tablespoons tomato passata

2 garlic cloves, minced

2 teaspoons thyme, chopped

½ teaspoon red pepper flakes

Directions:

Heat up a pot with the oil over medium heat, add the scallions, garlic and the pepper flakes and sauté for 5 minutes.

Add the chard and the other ingredients, toss, bring to a simmer and cook over medium heat for 30 minutes more.

Ladle the soup into bowls and serve for lunch.

Nutrition: calories 150, fat 8, fiber 2, carbs 4, protein 9

## 104. Hot Roasted Peppers Cream

Preparation time: 10 minutes

Cooking time: 30 minutes

Servings: 4

Ingredients:

1 red chili pepper, minced

4 garlic cloves, minced

2 pounds mixed bell peppers, roasted, peeled and chopped

4 scallions, chopped

1 cup coconut cream

Salt and black pepper to the taste

2 tablespoons olive oil

½ tablespoon basil, chopped

4 cups vegetable stock

¼ cup chives, chopped

Directions:

Heat up a pot with the oil over medium heat, add the garlic and the chili pepper and sauté for 5 minutes.

Add the peppers and the other ingredients, toss, bring to a simmer and cook over medium heat for 25 minutes.

Blend the soup using an immersion blender, divide into bowls and serve.

Nutrition: calories 140, fat 2, fiber 2, carbs 5, protein 8

## 105. Eggplant and Peppers Soup

Preparation time: 10 minutes

Cooking time: 40 minutes

Servings: 4

Ingredients:

2 red bell peppers, chopped

3 scallions, chopped

3 garlic cloves, minced

2 tablespoon olive oil

Salt and black pepper to the taste

5 cups vegetable stock

1 bay leaf

½ cup coconut cream

1 pound eggplants, roughly cubed

2 tablespoons basil, chopped

Directions:

Heat up a pot with the oil over medium heat, add the scallions and the garlic and sauté for 5 minutes.

Add the peppers and the eggplants and sauté for 5 minutes more.

Add the remaining ingredients, toss, bring to a simmer, cook for 30 minutes, ladle into bowls and serve for lunch.

Nutrition: calories 180, fat 2, fiber 3, carbs 5, protein 10

## 106. Eggplant and Olives Stew

Preparation time: 10 minutes

Cooking time: 30 minutes

Servings: 4

Ingredients:

2 scallions, chopped

2 tablespoons avocado oil

2 garlic cloves, chopped

1 bunch parsley, chopped

Salt and black pepper to the taste

1 teaspoon basil, dried

1 teaspoon cumin, dried

2 eggplants, roughly cubed

1 cup green olives, pitted and sliced

3 tablespoons balsamic vinegar

½ cup tomato passata

Directions:

Heat up a pot with the oil over medium heat, add the scallions, garlic, basil and cumin and sauté for 5 minutes.

Add the eggplants and the other ingredients, toss, cook over medium heat for 25 minutes more, divide into bowls and serve.

Nutrition: calories 93, fat 1.8, fiber 10.6, carbs 18.6, protein 3.4

## 107. Cauliflower and Artichokes Soup

Preparation time: 10 minutes

Cooking time: 25 minutes

Servings: 4

Ingredients:

1 pound cauliflower florets

1 cup canned artichoke hearts, drained and chopped

2 scallions, chopped

2 tablespoons olive oil

2 garlic cloves, minced

6 cups vegetable stock

Salt and black pepper to the taste

2/3 cup coconut cream

2 tablespoons cilantro, chopped

Directions:

Heat up a pot with the oil over medium heat, add the scallions and the garlic and sauté for 5 minutes.

Add the cauliflower and the other ingredients, toss, bring to a simmer and cook over medium heat for 20 minutes more.

Blend the soup using an immersion blender, divide it into bowls and serve.

Nutrition: calories 207, fat 17.2, fiber 6.2, carbs 14.1, protein 4.7

# 108. Hot Cabbage Soup

Preparation time: 10 minutes

Cooking time: 30 minutes

Servings: 4

Ingredients:

3 spring onions, chopped

1 green cabbage head, shredded

2 tablespoons olive oil

1 tablespoon ginger, grated

1 teaspoon cumin, ground

6 cups vegetable stock

Salt and black pepper to the taste

1 teaspoon hot paprika

1 teaspoon chili powder

1 tablespoon cilantro, chopped

Directions:

Heat up a pot with the oil over medium heat, add the spring onions, ginger and the cumin and sauté for 5 minutes.

Add the cabbage and the other ingredients, stir, bring to a simmer and cook over medium heat for 25 minutes more.

Ladle the soup into bowls and serve for lunch.

Nutrition: calories 117, fat 7.5, fiber 5.2, carbs 12.7, protein 2.8

# 109. Macaroni with Mushrooms

 Preparation Time: 30 Minutes

Servings: 5

Ingredients:

1 pack : 17 ozmacaroni, egg-free

7 oz button mushrooms, chopped

1 large onion, finely chopped

1 large tomato, peeled and finely chopped

1 tbsp tomato paste

3 tbsp coconut oil, unsalted

1 tsp salt

¼ tsp freshly ground black pepper

1 tsp cayenne pepper

1 bay leaf

1 tbsp vegetable oil

Directions:

Plug in your instant pot and grease the steel cooking insert with one tablespoon of vegetable oil. Press "Sautee" button and add finely chopped onion. Cook until translucent, stirring constantly.

Now, add finely chopped tomato, tomato paste, coconut oil, salt, black pepper, and cayenne pepper. Continue to cook until tomato completely softens, stirring occasionally.

Now, add mushrooms and one cup of water. Give it a good stir and close the lid. Set the steam release handle and press the "Manual" button. Cook for 5 minutes on high pressure. When done, perform a quick release and open the cooker. Remove everything from the pot.

Place the macaroni in your steel insert and add 2 cups of water. Close the lid and press the "Manual" button. Set the timer for 4 minutes. After you hear the end signal, perform a quick release to open the cooker. Transfer macaroni to a large bowl, and top with mushroom mixture.

Serve immediately.

# 110. Broccoli Orecchiette

Preparation Time: 25 Minutes

Servings: 4

Ingredients:

1 pack : 8ozvegan orecchiette

1 lb broccoli, roughly chopped

2 garlic cloves

3 tbsp of extra virgin olive oil

1 cup of grated tofu

1 tsp of salt

¼ tsp of pepper

Directions:

Place the orecchiette pasta and broccoli in your instant pot. Add enough water to cover and securely lock the lid. Set the timer for 10 minutes in the "Manual" mode.

When done, press "Cancel" and perform a quick release to release the cooker's pressure. Drain the broccoli and pasta. Set aside.

With the cooker's lid off, press "Sautee" and heat up the olive oil. Add garlic and stir-fry for 2-3 minutes. Now add broccoli, orecchiette, salt, and pepper. Stir well and cook for 2 more minutes.

Press the "Cancel" button and stir in the grated tofu.

Serve immediately.

## 111. Eggplant Lasagna

Preparation Time: 25 Minutes

Servings: 8

Ingredients:

1 large eggplant

1 package : 15 ounces tofu)

1 jar : 25 ounces marinara sauce )

1/2 cup cashews

1/2 cup nutritional yeast

3 cloves garlic

4 fresh basil leaves

1/2 teaspoon oregano

1/2 cup unsweetened nondairy milk

1 teaspoon salt

Pepper, to taste

Cooked pasta, for serving

Directions:

Peel the eggplant and cut it into thin slices.

Combine the cashews, yeast, tofu, nondairy milk, garlic, basil, and oregano in a food processor and pulse to make the ricotta.

Oil the instant pot and add a third of the marinara. Add a layer of eggplant, using half of it, followed by half of the ricotta. Repeat the layers and then top with the last of the sauce.

Seal the lid and cook on high for 3 minutes. Check the consistency – if it is too watery, switch the instant pot to the sauté setting and heat for a while with the lid off to evaporate some of the water.

Serve over pasta!

## 112. Lasagna with Pumpkin Ricotta

Preparation Time: 45 Minutes

Servings: 6

Ingredients:

15 ounces tofu

1 can white beans, drained and rinsed

1 can : 15 ouncescooked pumpkin

10 ounces whole wheat lasagna noodles

1 small jar sun-dried tomatoes in oil, drained

1/4 cup nutritional yeast

1/2 tablespoon oregano

1/4 teaspoon thyme

1/2 teaspoon parsley

1/2 teaspoon dried basil

1 teaspoon onion powder

2 cloves garlic, minced

Salt and pepper, to taste

1 jar : 24 ouncesmarinara sauce

1 tablespoon olive oil

Directions:

Combine olive oil and sun-dried tomatoes in a food processor until smooth.

Add the tofu, pumpkin, garlic, yeast, and seasonings to the tomato mixture and process until creamy.

Spray the instant pot with nonstick spray, then pour in a thin layer of sauce.

Add a layer of the lasagna noodles, breaking them to make them fit in the instant pot.

Top with one-third of the ricotta, then one-third of the beans. Repeat the layers twice, then top with one last layer of lasagna noodles and sauce. Seal the lid and cook on high for 10 minutes. Let the pressure release naturally.

## 113. Smoked Double Cheese Macaroni

Preparation Time: 20 Minutes

Servings: 4

Ingredients:

8 ounces dried whole wheat macaroni

4 cups nondairy milk

2 tablespoons vegan chicken-flavored bouillon

2 cups shredded vegan cheddar cheese

1 cup shredded vegan mozzarella cheese

1/2 teaspoon liquid smoke

1/8 teaspoon paprika

1/2 teaspoon Cajun seasoning

Salt and pepper, to taste

Directions:

Add all the ingredients except for the cheese to the instant pot. Seal the lid and cook on low 4 minutes.

Let pressure release naturally, then remove the lid and stir in the cheese.

## 114. Mushroom Garlic Lasagna

Preparation Time: 45 Minutes

Servings: 4

Ingredients:

15 ounces tofu

10 ounces whole wheat lasagna noodles

20 ounces mushrooms, sliced

Juice of 1/2 lemon

3 cloves garlic

1/4 cup nutritional yeast

1 1/2 tablespoons vegan chicken-flavored bouillon

2 tablespoons olive oil

2 sprigs rosemary

1 cup water

1 teaspoon salt

Directions:

Combine the lemon juice, bouillon, yeast, tofu, water, garlic, and salt in a food processor and blend until smooth to make the sauce.

Add the oil, mushrooms, and rosemary to the instant pot and sauté for 10 minutes. Discard the rosemary and set aside the mushrooms.

Pour one-fifth of the sauce into the bottom of the instant pot, then add a layer of noodles. Break the lasagna noodles to make them fit. Add one-third of the mushrooms followed by another fifth of the sauce. Repeat the layers two more times, then end with a final layer of noodles and sauce.

Cook on high for 10 minutes and let pressure release naturally.

## 115. Simple Chicken Garlic Risotto

Preparation Time: 18 Minutes

Servings: 6

Ingredients:

1 cup Arborio rice

2 cups water

2 tablespoons vegan chicken-flavored bouillon

2 cloves garlic, minced

Salt and pepper, to taste

Directions:

Add the ingredients to the instant pot.

Seal the lid and cook for 8 minutes, letting the pressure release naturally.

Serve with green veggies.

## 116. Creamy Butternut Squash Risotto

Preparation Time: 20 Minutes

Servings: 6

Ingredients:

1 can : 15 ouncescooked butternut squash

1 cup Arborio rice

2 cups water

1/2 cup nutritional yeast

1/8 teaspoon nutmeg

1/8 teaspoon cinnamon

1 teaspoon thyme

1/8 teaspoon dried rosemary

Salt and pepper, to taste

Directions:

Add the ingredients to the instant pot and cook on high 8 minutes. Let the pressure release naturally.

## 117. Broccoli Cheddar Rice

Preparation Time: 30 Minutes

Servings: 6

Ingredients:

1-pound fresh broccoli

2 cups long-grain brown rice

2 1/2 cups water

1 cup shredded vegan cheddar cheese

3 tablespoons vegan chicken-flavored bouillon

1/2 cup nutritional yeast

1/4 teaspoon salt

1/4 teaspoon onion powder

1/4 teaspoon pepper

Directions:

Combine everything but the cheese in the instant pot. Seal the lid and cook on high 20 minutes, then let pressure release naturally.

Stir in the cheese and serve.

# 118. Buttercup Squash

Preparation Time: 45 Minutes

Servings: 6

Ingredients:

1 large kabocha or buttercup squash

2 cups cooked brown rice

1½ cups cooked pinto beans or 1 : 15-ouncecan beans, rinsed and drained

1 cup fresh or thawed frozen corn kernels

1 medium-size yellow onion, minced

2 garlic cloves, minced

1 minced chipotle chile in adobo

2 teaspoons olive oil : optional

1 teaspoon ground cumin

1 teaspoon ground coriander

1 teaspoon dried thyme

2 tablespoons minced fresh flat-leaf parsley

Salt and freshly ground black pepper

Directions:

Chop the top off your squash so it will fit in your instant pot and scoop out the seeds. Chop the bottom so it sits nicely.

Heat the oil in your instant pot with the lid off.

Add the onion and soften for 5 minutes.

Stir in the garlic, chile, cumin, thyme, and coriander, heat another minute, then remove and put in a bowl.

Add the beans, rice, corn, parsley, salt and pepper.

Pack the stuffing into your squash and put the squash in the instant pot.

Pour hot water in so it comes up an inch of the way up your squash.

Seal and cook on Meat for 35 minutes.

Release the pressure quickly and serve.

# 119. Quinoa with Mushrooms

Preparation Time: 30 Minutes

Servings: 3

Ingredients:

1 cup quinoa

1 cup button mushrooms, sliced

1 cup cherry tomatoes, halved

1 cup vegetable stock

2 garlic cloves, finely chopped

1 medium-sized onion, finely chopped

1 medium-sized carrot, sliced

2 tbsp olive oil

1 tbsp lemon juice, freshly squeezed

1 tsp salt

¼ tsp black pepper, freshly ground

Directions:

Plug in your instant pot and press "Sautee" button. Grease the stainless steel insert with some olive oil. Add onions and garlic and stir-fry for 3 minutes.

Add carrots and mushrooms and cook for 5 minutes, stirring occasionally.

Sprinkle with lemon juice, salt, and pepper to taste.

Add the remaining ingredients and seal the lid. Press the "Manual" button and adjust the steam release handle. Set the timer for 15 minutes and cook on high pressure.

When done, press "Cancel" button and turn off the pot. Release the pressure naturally. Let it stand covered for 10 minutes before opening.

Serve warm.

## 120. Mushroom Spicy Quinoa

Preparation Time: 6 Minutes

Servings: 4-6

Ingredients:

1cup chopped mushrooms

1: 4-ouncecan diced green chilies, chopped

1teaspoon vegan Worcestershire sauce

1small yellow onion, minced

1cup quinoa, rinsed and drained

2garlic cloves, minced

Salt and black pepper

1teaspoon dried thyme

3cups cooked black-eyed peas

1½cups vegetable broth

1teaspoon smoked paprika

1: 14.5-ouncecan diced tomatoes, chopped

Directions:

In your instant pot add the mushrooms, chilies, sauce, onion, quinoa, garlic, seasoning, tomatoes, paprika, broth, thyme and black eyed peas.

Mix well and cover.

Cook for about 5 minutes.

Serve hot.

# 121. Cheesy Vegetable Risotto

Preparation Time: 10 Minutes

Servings: 4

Ingredients:

¼ cup grated vegan Parmesan cheese

1¼cups Arborio rice

2teaspoons olive oil : optional

2cups canned artichoke hearts, chopped

3cups vegetable broth

½teaspoon salt

1teaspoon dried thyme

¼cup dry white wine

Black pepper

2shallots, minced

2teaspoons fresh lemon juice

Directions:

In your instant pot add the oil and toss the shallots and artichoke hearts for 1 minute.

Add in the seasoning, white wine, thyme, lemon juice, broth, rice and cheese.

Mix well and add the lid.

Cook for about 8 minutes.

Serve hot.

## 122. Mushroom Garlic Polenta

 Preparation Time: 6 Minutes

Servings: 6

Ingredients:

1pound mushrooms, sliced

7cups boiling vegetable broth

1½cups coarse-ground polenta

3garlic cloves, minced

Salt and black pepper

2teaspoons olive oil

3cups marinara sauce

Directions:

In your instant pot add the polenta.

Add the mushroom, broth, garlic, seasoning, oil and sauce.

Mix well and cover with lid.

Cook for about 5 minutes.

Serve hot.

## 123. Barley, Carrot & Mushroom Stew

 Preparation Time: 8 Minutes

Servings: 4

Ingredients:

3cups vegetable broth

1large carrot, minced

¾cup fresh frozen peas

1onion, minced

¼cup dry white wine

3garlic cloves, minced

1cup pearl barley

1small celery rib, minced

½small red bell pepper, seeded and minced

1teaspoon minced fresh thyme

6ounces mushrooms, chopped

1½cups cooked cannellini beans

Salt and black pepper

Directions:

In your instant pot add all the vegetables.

Add the mushroom, beans, seasoning, herbs and spices.

Add the barley, white wine, and broth.

Mix well and cover.

Cook for about 8 minutes.

Serve hot.

## 124. Sweet Potato Grits Curry

 Preparation Time: 6 Minutes

Servings: 6

Ingredients:

4½cups vegetable broth

4scallions, minced

1½cups stone-ground grits

1large sweet potatoes, peeled and diced

4 green chilies, diced

Salt and black pepper

Directions:

Add the broth, sweet potato, grits, scallions, green chilies and seasoning in your instant pot.

Mix well and add the lid.

Cook for about 5 minutes.

Serve hot.

# 125. Peppers Stuffed With Quinoa

Preparation Time: 30 Minutes

Servings: 4

These peppers combine a lot of strong tastes for a South American medley that is truly delightful.

Ingredients:

4 large bell peppers : any color or a combination

2 cups cooked quinoa

1 cup thawed frozen baby green peas

½ cup chopped fresh flat-leaf parsley leaves

⅓ cup minced oil-packed sun-dried tomatoes

1 : 8-ouncejar marinated artichoke hearts, drained and chopped

1 large red onion, minced

½ teaspoon dried marjoram

2 teaspoons olive oil : optional

2 teaspoons freshly squeezed lemon juice

 Salt and freshly ground black pepper

Directions:

Top and hollow the peppers. Take the stems off and dice the rest of the top.

Warm the oil in your instant pot with the lid off.

When hot, add the onion and soften for 5 minutes.

Add the pepper tops and cook another 3 minutes.

Add the tomatoes and marjoram.

Put the mix in a bowl and add the artichokes, peas, quinoa, lemon, parsley, and salt and pepper.

Pack the stuffing into the peppers and put them in the steamer basket of your instant pot.

Put a cup of water in your instant pot. Lower the steamer basket.

Seal and cook on Steam for 24 minutes.

Depressurize naturally and serve immediately.

# 126. Rice-Stuffed Winter Squash

Preparation Time: 40 Minutes

Servings: 4

Ingredients:

1 large kabocha or buttercup squash

1 large yellow onion, minced

2 celery ribs, minced

1 carrot, peeled and minced

2 garlic cloves, minced

2 tablespoons tomato paste

2 cups cooked rice, couscous, or quinoa

1 cup chopped dried apricots or golden raisins

½ cup hot water

½ cup chopped toasted slivered almonds

¼ cup minced fresh flat-leaf parsley leaves

2 teaspoons olive oil : optional

1½ teaspoons ground coriander

1 teaspoon dried thyme

1 teaspoon ground cinnamon

½ teaspoon ground allspice

½ teaspoon paprika

¼ teaspoon cayenne pepper

1 tablespoon freshly squeezed lemon juice

Salt and freshly ground black pepper

Directions:

Chop the top off your squash so it will fit in your instant pot and scoop out the seeds. Chop the bottom so it sits nicely.

Heat the oil in your instant pot with the lid off.

Add the onion, carrots, garlic, and celery and soften for 5 minutes.

Stir in the tomato paste, coriander, thyme, cinnamon, paprika, cayenne, and allspice, heat another minute, then remove and put in a bowl.

Add the apricots, almonds, rice, parsley, lemon juice, salt and pepper.

Pack the stuffing into your squash and put the squash in the instant pot.

Pour hot water in so it comes up an inch of the way up your squash.

Seal and cook on Meat for 35 minutes.

Release the pressure quickly and serve.

# 127. Bulgur-Stuffed Eggplant

Preparation Time: 35 Minutes

Servings: 4

Ingredients:

1 large eggplant

1½ cups cooked dark red kidney beans or 1 : 15-ouncecan beans, rinsed and drained

1 cup cooked bulgur

1 small onion, minced

½ small green bell pepper, seeded and minced

1 small celery rib, minced

4 garlic cloves, minced

1 jalapeño chile, seeded and minced

1 chipotle chile in adobo, finely minced

1 : 14.5-ouncecan crushed tomatoes

1 tablespoon chili powder

2 teaspoons olive oil : optional

1 teaspoon dried basil

1 teaspoon dried thyme

 Salt and freshly ground black pepper

Directions:

Halve the eggplants and scoop out the flesh, leaving ¼ an inch of shell.

Chop up the scooped eggplant.

Warm the oil in your instant pot.

Add the onion, celery, garlic, bell pepper, chopped eggplant, jalapeno, and thyme and cook for 5 minutes.

Put the onion mix in a bowl and add the beans, bulgur, and chipotle chile. Season with salt stnd pepper and mix.

Fill the eggplants with the stuffing and place in your instant pot.

In a bowl mix tomatoes, chili powder, basil, and salt and pepper.

Pour the tomatoes over the eggplants. Seal and cook on Stew for 25 minutes.

Depressurize quickly and serve.

# 128. Rice with Vegan Bacon

Preparation Time: 18 Minutes

Servings: 4

Ingredients:

2 cups basmati rice

1 cup vegan bacon, sliced

1 medium onion, finely chopped

½ cup green peas

3 tbsp extra virgin olive oil

3 garlic cloves, finely chopped

1 tsp dried thyme

1 tsp salt

4 cups of vegetable broth

Directions:

Plug in your instant pot and press "Sautee" button. Grease the stainless steel insert and add onions and garlic. Stir-fry for 3-4 minutes, or until translucent.

Add all the remaining ingredients and close the lid. Adjust the steam release handle and press "Manual" button. Set the timer for 5 minutes and cook on high pressure.

When done, press "Cancel" button and turn off the pot. Release the pressure naturally.

Transfer to a serving dish and stir well before serving.

Enjoy!

# 129. Southwestern Quinoa

Preparation Time: 15 Minutes

Servings: 8

Ingredients:

1 cup quinoa

2 tablespoons olive oil

1 shallot, chopped

2 tablespoons tomato paste

1 bell pepper, chopped

2 tablespoons vegan chicken-flavored bouillon

2 cloves garlic, minced

1 teaspoon salt

1/8 teaspoon coriander

1/2 teaspoon chili powder

1/2 teaspoon cumin

1 1/2 cups water

Directions:

Heat the olive oil on the sauté setting and cook the shallot for 5 minutes. Add the garlic and bell pepper and cook for 5 more minutes.

Add the rest of the ingredients to the instant pot, seal the lid, and cook on high for 1 minute, then let pressure release naturally.

## 130. Instant Basmati Rice

Preparation Time: 15 Minutes

Servings: 8

Ingredients:

2 cups water

2 cups brown basmati rice

1/4 teaspoon salt

Directions:

Spray your instant pot with oil and combine the water, rice, and salt inside making sure to leave room below the fill line.

Seal the lid and cook on high for 4 minutes.

# 131. Black Beans and Brown Rice Recipe

Preparation Time: 55 Minutes

Servings: 2

Ingredients:

1/2 cup dry black beans

1 cup brown rice : or brown rice medley, if available

2 1/2 cups water

1/2 red pepper, diced

1/2 red onion, diced

2 garlic cloves, minced

1 tsp vegetable base or a bouillon cube

1/2 tsp cayenne pepper

1 tbsp chili powder

1 tsp cumin

Directions:

Add garlic and onion to Instant Pot along with 1/2 cup water and Switch on 'Sautée' button. Allow it to sautée for about 5 minutes. Switch on 'Keep Warm/Cancel' button.

Except for red pepper, add rest of ingredients to Instant Pot. Cover the Pot with lid and set steam release handle to 'sealing'. Put the lid on top. Switch on manual button and set the timer to 25 minutes over high pressure.

Once done, let pressure release naturally for 10-15 minutes. Set steam release handle to 'venting' to release remaining steam. Open the lid.

Add diced red pepper and serve.

## 132. Sweet Zucchini Cornbread

Preparation Time: 40 Minutes

Servings: 1 LOAF

Ingredients:

1/2 cup frozen corn kernels

1/4 cup shredded zucchini

1/2 tablespoon apple cider vinegar

1/4 cup nondairy milk

1 cup cornmeal

1/2 teaspoon sugar

1/2 teaspoon maple syrup

1/4 teaspoon salt

3/4 teaspoon baking powder

1/4 teaspoon baking soda

1/2 tablespoon ground flaxseed

1 1/2 tablespoons warm water

Directions:

Mix the milk and vinegar in a small bowl and let it rest for 5 minutes.

Meanwhile, combine the warm water with the flaxseed.

Mix together the salt, baking powder and soda, and cornmeal before adding the vinegar mixture, moistened flaxseed, corn, zucchini, and pepper. If the mixture is too dry, add more water a teaspoon at a time.

Spray a 16-ounce coffee can with nonstick spray. Set it on top of a rack in the instant pot, and pour water into the pot until half of the coffee can is submerged. Spray a piece of foil with nonstick spray and cover the top of the coffee can. The foil should allow extra room for the bread to grow as it cooks. Make sure it is sealed tightly around the mouth of the can by using a piece of cooking twine.

Seal the lid on the instant pot and cook on high for 25 minutes before letting the pressure release naturally. After you remove the lid, use a toothpick to double check that the bread is done.

Serve with beans or spicy chili!

# 133. Sweet Berry Maple Cornbread

Preparation Time: 40 Minutes

Servings: 2 LOAVES

Ingredients:

6 ounces fresh strawberries, chopped

6 ounces fresh blueberries

1 cup cornmeal

1 cup whole wheat pastry flour

1/2 teaspoon salt

1 1/2 teaspoons baking powder

1/2 teaspoon baking soda

5 tablespoons maple syrup

6 ounces nondairy yogurt

3 tablespoons olive oil

1 tablespoon ground flaxseed

3 tablespoons warm water

Directions:

Mix together the dry ingredients.

In a separate bowl, combine the flaxseed and warm water, then add the yogurt, maple syrup, oil, and strawberries.

Add the wet ingredients to the dry and mix well. Add additional water 1 teaspoon at a time if needed.

Spray the first 16-ounce coffee can with nonstick spray. Set it on top of a rack in the instant pot, and pour water into the pot until half of the coffee can is submerged. Spray a piece of foil with nonstick spray and cover the top of the coffee can. The foil should allow extra room for the bread to grow as it cooks. Make sure it is sealed tightly around the mouth of the can by using a piece of cooking twine.

Seal the lid on the instant pot and cook on high for 25 minutes before letting the pressure release naturally. After you remove the lid, use a toothpick to double check that the bread is done. This recipe will yield enough for two can sized loafs; repeat the process if you desire two loafs, or cut the recipe in half for just one loaf.

# 134. Autumn Pumpkin Bread

Preparation Time: 40 Minutes

Servings: 1 LOAF

Ingredients:

1/2 cup pumpkin purée

1/4 cup maple syrup

1/4 cup molasses

2 tablespoon olive oil

1/2 teaspoon vanilla extract

1/4 teaspoon baking soda

1 cup whole wheat pastry flour

1/2 tablespoon baking powder

1/4 teaspoon ground cloves

3/4 tablespoon ground ginger

1/2 teaspoon cinnamon

1/8 teaspoon nutmeg

1/4 teaspoon allspice

1/8 teaspoon chili powder

1/8 teaspoon salt

1 tablespoon ground flaxseed

1 tablespoons water

Directions:

Combine the flaxseed and water.

In a separate bowl, combine the dry ingredients. Add the flaxseed mixture to rest of the wet ingredients, then combine with the dry ingredients.

Spray a 16-ounce coffee can with nonstick spray. Set it on top of a rack in the instant pot, and pour water into the pot until half of the coffee can is submerged. Spray a piece of foil with nonstick spray and cover the top of the coffee can. The foil should allow extra room for the bread to grow as it cooks. Make sure it is sealed tightly around the mouth of the can by using a piece of cooking twine.

Seal the lid on the instant pot and cook on high for 25 minutes before letting the pressure release naturally. After you remove the lid, use a toothpick to double check that the bread is done.

## 135. Herbed Orange Bread

Preparation Time: 40 Minutes

Servings: 1 LOAF

Ingredients:

1 cup whole wheat pastry flour

1/4 cup orange juice

1/2 tablespoon lemon juice

1/2 teaspoon lemon zest

1/2 teaspoon vanilla extract

1/2 teaspoon almond extract

1/4 cup sugar

1/4 teaspoon baking soda

1/2 tablespoon baking powder

1/2 tablespoon ground flaxseed

1/4 tablespoon minced fresh rosemary

1 tablespoon water

1/4 cup applesauce

1 tablespoons olive oil

Directions:

Combine the flaxseed and water.

In a separate bowl, combine the dry ingredients. Add the flaxseed mixture to rest of the wet ingredients, then combine with the dry ingredients.

Spray a 16-ounce coffee can with nonstick spray. Set it on top of a rack in the instant pot, and pour water into the pot until half of the coffee can is submerged. Spray a piece of foil with nonstick spray and cover the top of the coffee can. The foil should allow extra room for the bread to grow as it cooks. Make sure it is sealed tightly around the mouth of the can by using a piece of cooking twine.

Seal the lid on the instant pot and cook on high for 25 minutes before letting the pressure release naturally. After you remove the lid, use a toothpick to double check that the bread is done.

# 136. Walnut  & Chocolate Chip Banana Bread

Preparation Time: 40 Minutes

Servings: 1 LOAF

Ingredients:

1 1/2 banana, mashed

1/4 cup chocolate chips

1/4 cup walnuts

1 cup whole wheat pastry flour

1/4 teaspoon baking soda

1/2 tablespoon baking powder

1 tablespoon ground flaxseed

2 tablespoon water

1/4 cup applesauce

1 tablespoon olive oil

1/4 cup sugar

1/2 teaspoon vanilla extract

Directions:

In a separate bowl, combine the dry ingredients. Combine the wet ingredients in another bowl, then add to the dry ingredients and mix well. Stir in the chocolate chips.

Spray a 16-ounce coffee can with nonstick spray. Set it on top of a rack in the instant pot, and pour water into the pot until half of the coffee can is submerged. Spray a piece of foil with nonstick spray and cover the top of the coffee can. The foil should allow extra room for the bread to grow as it cooks. Make sure it is sealed tightly around the mouth of the can by using a piece of cooking twine.

Seal the lid on the instant pot and cook on high for 25 minutes before letting the pressure release naturally. After you remove the lid, use a toothpick to double check that the bread is done.

# Chapter 5.Dinner recipes

### 137.Classic Black Beans Chili

Preparation time: 10 minutes

Cooking time: 3 hours

Servings: 4

Ingredients:

½ cup quinoa

2 and ½ cups veggie stock

14 ounces canned tomatoes, chopped

15 ounces canned black beans, drained

¼ cup green bell pepper, chopped

¼ cup red bell pepper, chopped

A pinch of salt and black pepper

2 garlic cloves, minced

1 carrots, shredded

1 small chili pepper, chopped

2 teaspoons chili powder

1 teaspoon cumin, ground

A pinch of cayenne pepper

½ cup corn

1 teaspoon oregano, dried

For the vegan sour cream:

A drizzle of apple cider vinegar

4 tablespoons water

½ cup cashews, soaked overnight and drained

1 teaspoon lime juice

Directions:

Put the stock in your slow cooker.

Add quinoa, tomatoes, beans, red and green bell pepper, garlic, carrot, salt, pepper, corn, cumin, cayenne, chili powder, chili pepper and oregano, stir, cover and cook on High for 3 hours.

Meanwhile, put the cashews in your blender.

Add water, vinegar and lime juice and pulse really well.

Divide beans chili into bowls, top with vegan sour cream and serve.

Enjoy!

Nutrition: calories 300, fat 4, fiber 4, carbs 10, protein 7

## 138. Amazing Potato Dish

Preparation time: 10 minutes

Cooking time: 3 hours

Servings: 4

Ingredients:

1 and ½ pounds potatoes, peeled and roughly chopped

1 tablespoon olive oil

3 tablespoons water

1 small yellow onion, chopped

½ cup veggie stock cube, crumbled

½ teaspoon coriander, ground

½ teaspoon cumin, ground

½ teaspoon garam masala

½ teaspoon chili powder

Black pepper to the taste

½ pound spinach, roughly torn

Directions:

Put the potatoes in your slow cooker.

Add oil, water, onion, stock cube, coriander, cumin, garam masala, chili powder, black pepper and spinach.

Stir, cover and cook on High for 3 hours.

Divide into bowls and serve.

Enjoy!

Nutrition: calories 270, fat 4, fiber 6, carbs 8, protein 12

## 139. Textured Sweet Potatoes and Lentils Delight

Preparation time: 10 minutes

Cooking time: 4 hours and 30 minutes

Servings: 6

Ingredients:

6 cups sweet potatoes, peeled and cubed

2 teaspoons coriander, ground

2 teaspoons chili powder

1 yellow onion, chopped

3 cups veggie stock

4 garlic cloves, minced

A pinch of sea salt and black pepper

10 ounces canned coconut milk

1 cup water

1 and ½ cups red lentils

Directions:

Put sweet potatoes in your slow cooker.

Add coriander, chili powder, onion, stock, garlic, salt and pepper, stir, cover and cook on High for 3 hours.

Add lentils, stir, cover and cook for 1 hour and 30 minutes.

Add water and coconut milk, stir well, divide into bowls and serve right away.

Enjoy!

Nutrition: calories 300, fat 10, fiber 8, carbs 16, protein 10

## 140. Incredibly Tasty Pizza

Preparation time: 1 hour and 10 minutes

Cooking time: 1 hour and 45 minutes

Servings: 3

Ingredients:

For the dough:

½ teaspoon Italian seasoning

1 and ½ cups whole wheat flour

1 and ½ teaspoons instant yeast

1 tablespoon olive oil

A pinch of salt

½ cup warm water

Cooking spray

For the sauce:

¼ cup green olives, pitted and sliced

¼ cup kalamata olives, pitted and sliced

½ cup tomatoes, crushed

1 tablespoon parsley, chopped

1 tablespoon capers, rinsed

¼ teaspoon garlic powder

¼ teaspoon basil, dried

¼ teaspoon oregano, dried

¼ teaspoon palm sugar

¼ teaspoon red pepper flakes

A pinch of salt and black pepper

½ cup cashew mozzarella, shredded

Directions:

In your food processor, mix yeast with Italian seasoning, a pinch of salt and flour.

Add oil and the water and blend well until you obtain a dough.

Transfer dough to a floured working surface, knead well, transfer to a greased bowl, cover and leave aside for 1 hour.

Meanwhile, in a bowl, mix green olives with kalamata olives, tomatoes, parsley, capers, garlic powder, oregano, sugar, salt, pepper and pepper flakes and stir well.

Transfer pizza dough to a working surface again and flatten it.

Shape so it will fit your slow cooker.

Grease your slow cooker with cooking spray and add dough.

Press well on the bottom.

Spread the sauce mix all over, cover and cook on High for 1 hour and 15 minutes.

Spread vegan mozzarella all over, cover again and cook on High for 30 minutes more.

Leave your pizza to cool down before slicing and serving it.

Nutrition: calories 340, fat 5, fiber 7, carbs 13, protein 15

## 141. Rich Beans Soup

Preparation time: 10 minutes

Cooking time: 7 hours

Servings: 4

Ingredients:

1 pound navy beans

1 yellow onion, chopped

4 garlic cloves, crushed

2 quarts veggie stock

A pinch of sea salt

Black pepper to the taste

2 potatoes, peeled and cubed

2 teaspoons dill, dried

1 cup sun-dried tomatoes, chopped

1 pound carrots, sliced

4 tablespoons parsley, minced

Directions:

Put the stock in your slow cooker.

Add beans, onion, garlic, potatoes, tomatoes, carrots, dill, salt and pepper, stir, cover and cook on Low for 7 hours.

Stir your soup, add parsley, divide into bowls and serve.

Enjoy!

Nutrition: calories 250, fat 4, fiber 3, carbs 9, protein 10

## 142. Delicious Baked Beans

Preparation time: 10 minutes

Cooking time: 12 hours

Servings: 8

Ingredients:

1 pound navy beans, soaked overnight and drained

1 cup maple syrup

1 cup bourbon

1 cup vegan bbq sauce

1 cup palm sugar

¼ cup ketchup

1 cup water

¼ cup mustard

¼ cup blackstrap molasses

¼ cup apple cider vinegar

¼ cup olive oil

2 tablespoons coconut aminos

Directions:

Put the beans in your slow cooker.

Add maple syrup, bourbon, bbq sauce, sugar, ketchup, water, mustard, molasses, vinegar, oil and coconut aminos.

Stir everything, cover and cook on Low for 12 hours.

Divide into bowls and serve.

Enjoy!

Nutrition: calories 430, fat 7, fiber 8, carbs 15, protein 19

## 143. Indian Lentils

Preparation time: 10 minutes

Cooking time: 3 hours

Servings: 4

Ingredients:

1 yellow bell pepper, chopped

1 sweet potato, chopped

2 and ½ cups lentils, already cooked

4 garlic cloves, minced

1 yellow onion, chopped

2 teaspoons cumin, ground

15 ounces canned tomato sauce

½ teaspoon ginger, ground

A pinch of cayenne pepper

1 tablespoons coriander, ground

1 teaspoon turmeric, ground

2 teaspoons paprika

2/3 cup veggie stock

1 teaspoon garam masala

A pinch of sea salt

Black pepper to the taste

Juice of 1 lemon

Directions:

Put the stock in your slow cooker.

Add potato, lentils, onion, garlic, cumin, bell pepper, tomato sauce, salt, pepper, ginger, coriander, turmeric, paprika, cayenne, garam masala and lemon juice.

Stir, cover and cook on High for 3 hours.

Stir your lentils mix again, divide into bowls and serve.

Enjoy!

Nutrition: calories 300, fat 6, fiber 5, carbs 9, protein 12

## 144. Delicious Butternut Squash Soup

Preparation time: 10 minutes

Cooking time: 6 hours

Servings: 8

Ingredients:

1 apple, cored, peeled and chopped

½ pound carrots, chopped

1 pound butternut squash, peeled and cubed

1 yellow onion, chopped

A pinch of sea salt

Black pepper to the taste

1 bay leaf

3 cups veggie stock

14 ounces canned coconut milk

¼ teaspoon sage, dried

Directions:

Put the stock in your slow cooker.

Add apple squash, carrots, onion, salt, pepper and bay leaf.

Stir, cover and cook on Low for 6 hours.

Transfer to your blender, add coconut milk and sage and pulse really well.

Ladle into bowls and serve right away.

Enjoy!

Nutrition: calories 200, fat 3, fiber 6, carbs 8, protein 10

## 145. Amazing Mushroom Stew

Preparation time: 10 minutes

Cooking time: 8 hours

Servings: 4

Ingredients:

2 garlic cloves, minced

1 celery stalk, chopped

1 yellow onion, chopped

1 and ½ cups firm tofu, pressed and cubed

1 cup water

10 ounces mushrooms, chopped

1 pound mixed peas, corn and carrots

2 and ½ cups veggie stock

1 teaspoon thyme, dried

2 tablespoons coconut flour

A pinch of sea salt

Black pepper to the taste

Directions:

Put the water and stock in your slow cooker.

Add garlic, onion, celery, mushrooms, mixed veggies, tofu, thyme, salt, pepper and flour.

Stir everything, cover and cook on Low for 8 hours.

Divide into bowls and serve hot.

Enjoy!

Nutrition: calories 230, fat 4, fiber 6, carbs 10, protein 7

## 146. Simple Tofu Dish

Preparation time: 10 minutes

Cooking time: 3 hours

Servings: 6

Ingredients:

1 big tofu package, cubed

1 tablespoon sesame oil

¼ cup pineapple, cubed

1 tablespoon olive oil

2 garlic cloves, minced

1 tablespoons brown rice vinegar

2 teaspoon ginger, grated

¼ cup soy sauce

5 big zucchinis, cubed

¼ cup sesame seeds

Directions:

In your food processor, mix sesame oil with pineapple, olive oil, garlic, ginger, soy sauce and vinegar and whisk well.

Add this to your slow cooker and mix with tofu cubes.

Cover and cook on High for 2 hours and 45 minutes.

Add sesame seeds and zucchinis, stir gently, cover and cook on High for 15 minutes.

Divide between plates and serve.

Enjoy!

Nutrition: calories 200, fat 3, fiber 4, carbs 9, protein 10

## 147. Special Jambalaya

Preparation time: 10 minutes

Cooking time: 6 hours

Servings: 4

Ingredients:

6 ounces soy chorizo, chopped

1 and ½ cups celery ribs, chopped

1 cup okra

1 green bell pepper, chopped

16 ounces canned tomatoes and green chilies, chopped

2 garlic cloves, minced

½ teaspoon paprika

1 and ½ cups veggie stock

A pinch of cayenne pepper

Black pepper to the taste

A pinch of salt

3 cups already cooked wild rice for serving

Directions:

Heat up a pan over medium high heat, add soy chorizo, stir, brown for a few minutes and transfer to your slow cooker.

Also, add celery, bell pepper, okra, tomatoes and chilies, garlic, paprika, salt, pepper and cayenne to your slow cooker.

Stir everything, add veggie stock, cover the slow cooker and cook on Low for 6 hours.

Divide rice on plates, top each serving with your vegan jambalaya and serve hot.

Enjoy!

Nutrition: calories 150, fat 3, fiber 7, carbs 15, protein 9

# 148. Delicious Chard Soup

Preparation time: 10 minutes

Cooking time: 8 hours

Servings: 6

Ingredients:

1 yellow onion, chopped

1 tablespoon olive oil

1 celery stalk, chopped

2 garlic cloves, minced

1 carrot, chopped

1 bunch Swiss chard, torn

1 cup brown lentils, dried

5 potatoes, peeled and cubed

1 tablespoon soy sauce

Black pepper to the taste

A pinch of sea salt

6 cups veggie stock

Directions:

Heat up a big pan with the oil over medium high heat, add onion, celery, garlic, carrot and Swiss chard, stir, cook for a few minutes and transfer to your slow cooker.

Also, add lentils, potatoes, soy sauce, salt, pepper and stock to the slow cooker, stir, cover and cook on Low for 8 hours.

Divide into bowls and serve hot.

Enjoy!

Nutrition: calories 200, fat 4, fiber 5, carbs 9, protein 12

# 149. Chinese Tofu and Veggies

Preparation time: 10 minutes

Cooking time: 4 hours

Servings: 4

Ingredients:

14 ounces extra firm tofu, pressed and cut into medium triangles

Cooking spray

2 teaspoons ginger, grated

1 yellow onion, chopped

3 garlic cloves, minced

8 ounces tomato sauce

¼ cup hoisin sauce

¼ teaspoon coconut aminos

2 tablespoons rice wine vinegar

1 tablespoon soy sauce

1 tablespoon spicy mustard

¼ teaspoon red pepper, crushed

2 teaspoons molasses

2 tablespoons water

A pinch of black pepper

3 broccoli stalks

1 green bell pepper, cut into squares

2 zucchinis, cubed

Directions:

Heat up a pan over medium high heat, add tofu pieces, brown them for a few minutes and transfer to your slow cooker.

Heat up the pan again over medium high heat, add ginger, onion, garlic and tomato sauce, stir, sauté for a few minutes and transfer to your slow cooker as well.

Add hoisin sauce, aminos, vinegar, soy sauce, mustard, red pepper, molasses, water and black pepper, stir gently, cover and cook on High for 3 hours.

Add zucchinis, bell pepper and broccoli, cover and cook on High for 1 more hour.

Divide between plates and serve right away.

Enjoy!

Nutrition: calories 300, fat 4, fiber 8, carbs 14, protein 13

# 150. Wonderful Corn Chowder

Preparation time: 10 minutes

Cooking time: 8 hours and 30 minutes

Servings: 6

Ingredients:

2 cups yellow onion, chopped

2 tablespoons olive oil

1 red bell pepper, chopped

1 pound gold potatoes, cubed

1 teaspoon cumin, ground

4 cups corn kernels

4 cups veggie stock

1 cup almond milk

A pinch of salt

A pinch of cayenne pepper

½ teaspoon smoked paprika

Chopped scallions for serving

Directions:

Heat up a pan with the oil over medium heat, add onion, stir and sauté for 5 minutes and then transfer to your slow cooker.

Add bell pepper, 1 cup corn, potatoes, paprika, cumin, salt and cayenne, stir, cover and cook on Low for 8 hours.

Blend this using an immersion blender and then mix with almond milk and the rest of the corn.

Stir chowder, cover and cook on Low for 30 minutes more.

Ladle into bowls and serve with chopped scallions on top.

Enjoy!

Nutrition: calories 200, fat 4, fiber 7, carbs 13, protein 16

# 151. Black Eyed Peas Stew

Preparation time: 10 minutes

Cooking time: 4 hours

Servings: 8

Ingredients:

3 celery stalks, chopped

2 carrots, sliced

1 yellow onion, chopped

1 sweet potato, cubed

1 green bell pepper, chopped

3 cups black-eyed peas, soaked for 8 hours and drained

1 cup tomato puree

4 cups veggie stock

A pinch of salt

Black pepper to the taste

1 chipotle chile, minced

1 teaspoon ancho chili powder

1 teaspoons sage, dried and crumbled

2 teaspoons cumin, ground

Chopped coriander for serving

Directions:

Put celery in your slow cooker.

Add carrots, onion, potato, bell pepper, black-eyed peas, tomato puree, salt, pepper, chili powder, sage, chili, cumin and stock.

Stir, cover and cook on High for 4 hours.

Stir stew again, divide into bowls and serve with chopped coriander on top.

Enjoy!

Nutrition: calories 200, fat 4, fiber 7, carbs 9, protein 16

# 152. White Bean Cassoulet

Preparation time: 10 minutes

Cooking time: 6 hours

Servings: 4

Ingredients:

2 celery stalks, chopped

3 leeks, sliced

4 garlic cloves, minced

2 carrots, chopped

2 cups veggie stock

15 ounces canned tomatoes, chopped

1 bay leaf

1 tablespoon Italian seasoning

30 ounces canned white beans, drained

For the breadcrumbs:

Zest from 1 lemon, grated

1 garlic clove, minced

2 tablespoons olive oil

1 cup vegan bread crumbs

¼ cup parsley, chopped

Directions:

Heat up a pan with a splash of the veggie stock over medium heat, add celery and leeks, stir and cook for 2 minutes.

Add carrots and garlic, stir and cook for 1 minute more.

Add this to your slow cooker and mix with stock, tomatoes, bay leaf, Italian seasoning and beans.

Stir, cover and cook on Low for 6 hours.

Meanwhile, heat up a pan with the oil over medium high heat, add bread crumbs, lemon zest, 1 garlic clove and parsley, stir and toast for a couple of minutes.

Divide your white beans mix into bowls, sprinkle bread crumbs mix on top and serve.

Enjoy!

Nutrition: calories 223, fat 3, fiber 7, carbs 10, protein 7

## 153. Light Jackfruit Dish

Preparation time: 10 minutes

Cooking time: 6 hours

Servings: 4

Ingredients:

40 ounces green jackfruit in brine, drained

½ cup agave nectar

½ cup gluten free tamari sauce

¼ cup soy sauce

1 cup white wine

2 tablespoons ginger, grated

8 garlic cloves, minced

1 pear, cored and chopped

1 yellow onion, chopped

½ cup water

4 tablespoons sesame oil

Directions:

Put jackfruit in your slow cooker.

Add agave nectar, tamari sauce, soy sauce, wine, ginger, garlic, pear, onion, water and oil.

Stir well, cover and cook on Low for 6 hours.

Divide jackfruit mix into bowls and serve.

Enjoy!

Nutrition: calories 160, fat 4, fiber 1, carbs 10, protein 3

## 154. Veggie Curry

Preparation time: 10 minutes

Cooking time: 4 hours

Servings: 4

Ingredients:

1 tablespoon ginger, grated

14 ounces canned coconut milk

Cooking spray

16 ounces firm tofu, pressed and cubed

1 cup veggie stock

¼ cup green curry paste

½ teaspoon turmeric

1 tablespoon coconut sugar

1 yellow onion, chopped

1 and ½ cup red bell pepper, chopped

A pinch of salt

¾ cup peas

1 eggplant, chopped

Directions:

Put the coconut milk in your slow cooker.

Add ginger, stock, curry paste, turmeric, sugar, onion, bell pepper, salt, peas and eggplant pieces, stir, cover and cook on High for 4 hours.

Meanwhile, spray a pan with cooking spray and heat up over medium high heat.

Add tofu pieces and brown them for a few minutes on each side.

Divide tofu into bowls, add slowly cooked curry mix on top and serve.

Enjoy!

Nutrition: calories 200, fat 4, fiber 6, carbs 10, protein 9

## 155. Banh Mi

Cooking Time: 20 minutes

Servings: 4

Ingredients

1 ½ cup raw vegetables, cabbage and carrots, shredded

1 cup hummus

8 oz. cooked tempeh, very finely sliced

1 long French baguette

½ small pack coriander leaves

½ small pack mint leaves

3 tablespoons white wine vinegar

1 teaspoon golden caster sugar

hot sauce

salt, to taste

Instructions

Place vegetables, vinegar, caster sugar and salt in a large bowl, mix well and set aside to marinate.

Heat the oven to 360F.

Place baguette in the oven pan, slice it in 4 slices, and cook in the oven for 5 minutes.

Once done, remove from the oven, spread hummus on 2 slices, top with 4 tempeh pieces and pickled vegetables.

Sprinkle coriander, mint leaves and top with the other 2 remaining baguette slices.

## 156. Sweet Potato Buddha Bowl Almond Butter Dressing

Cooking Time: 1 hour

Servings: 4

Ingredients

For the roasted vegetables:

1 large head broccoli, cut into florets

2 sweet potatoes, cubed

2 cloves garlic, minced

1 tablespoon toasted sesame oil

salt and pepper

For the mango coconut rice:

2 teaspoons coconut oil

1 cup unsweetened coconut milk

1 cup water

1 cup brown rice, uncooked

1 ripe mango, diced

For the almond butter dressing:

¼ cup natural creamy almond butter

4 tablespoons fresh orange juice

2 teaspoons maple syrup

½ teaspoon apple cider vinegar

1 teaspoon coconut oil, melted

Instructions

Place the pot over medium heat, add coconut oil.

Add brown rice and cook for 5 minutes, add water and coconut milk and bring it to a boil. Cover, reduce the heat and let it simmer for about 45 minutes.

When done add mango, salt, and set aside

Preheat the oven 375F and line a baking sheet with parchment paper.

Place sweet potatoes in a microwave safe bowl and heat it for about 4 minutes, then transfer to the prepared baking sheet.

Add broccoli florets, minced garlic to the baking sheet and mix well.

Bake in the oven for 30 minutes until tender.

Mix almond butter dressing ingredients in a medium bowl.

Serve rice in bowls, top with roasted vegetables and 2 tablespoons of the almond dressing.

## 157. Curry Spiced Sweet Potato Wild Rice Burgers

Cooking Time: 1 hour 15 minutes

Servings: 6

Ingredients

1 sweet potato

½ cup wild rice blend, uncooked

15 oz. can chickpeas, rinsed and drained

½ cup breadcrumbs

1/3 cup dried cranberries

2 teaspoons coconut oil

1 teaspoon curry powder

1 ½ teaspoons cumin

¼ teaspoon garlic powder

salt and pepper

Instructions

Prepare a pan with parchment lined paper and preheat the oven to 400F.

Place sweet potato on the pan and poke it with a fork. Bake for 45 minutes.

Place a small pan over medium heat. Add rice, water and bring to a boil. Cover, reduce the heat and let it simmer for 40 minutes.

Place sweet potato and chickpeas in a food processor, process for about 10 seconds and transfer to a large bowl.

Add cooked rice, curry powder, cumin, garlic, salt, pepper and mix well.

Add breadcrumbs, cranberries, pecans, mix well and scoop the mixture with damp hands and shape them into patties, set aside.

Place a large pan over medium heat, add coconut oil.

Fry patties in batches once oil is very hot for 8 minutes on each side.

## 158. Calabacitas Quesadillas

Cooking Time: 20 minutes

Servings: 2

Ingredients

2 large whole wheat tortillas

½ cup vegan Mexican shreds

½ onion, diced

1 jalapeno, seeded and diced

1 zucchini, quartered

kernels from 1 ear of sweet corn

1 teaspoon olive oil

2 cloves garlic, minced

¼ teaspoon cumin

salt and pepper

Instructions

Place a pan over medium heat. Add olive oil.

Add garlic, onion, jalapeno, zucchini, corn to the pan and cook for 6 minutes.

Season with cumin, salt and pepper. Set aside.

Return skillet to the medium heat, add oil.

Add wheat tortilla, onion-garlic mixture, top with vegetable shreds and cook tortilla for 3 minutes on each side until golden brown.

Remove from pan, cut into 4 pieces and serve with salsa and guacamole.

## 159. Chickpea Avocado Salad Sandwich With Cranberries

Cooking Time: 10 minutes

Servings: 2

Ingredients

15 oz. can chickpeas, rinsed and drained

¼ cup dried cranberries

1 large ripe avocado

4 slices gluten free bread, toasted

2 teaspoons freshly squeezed lemon juice

salt and pepper

Instructions

Combine chickpeas and avocado in a bowl, Mash until chunky in consistency.

Add lemon juice, cranberries, salt and pepper.

Spread the mixture on the toasted bread.

# 160. Rice Paper Rolls with Mango and Mint

Cooking Time: 20 minutes

Servings: 6

Ingredients

For the rice paper rolls:

6 sheets Vietnamese rice paper

1 cup fresh mint

3 cups lettuce, thinly sliced

1 ½ cups glass noodles, cooked

1 cup purple cabbage, thinly sliced

1 avocado, thinly sliced

1 cucumber, chopped

3 carrots, thinly sliced

1 mango, thinly sliced

3 green onions, cut into rings

6 radishes, thinly sliced

For the fried sesame tofu:

7 oz. block firm tofu, thinly sliced

1 teaspoon sesame oil

1 tablespoon soy sauce

1 tablespoon sesame seeds

For the peanut dipping sauce:

¼ cup chunky peanut butter

2 teaspoons soy sauce

1 clove of garlic, minced

4 tablespoons warm water

½ teaspoons Sriracha sauce

Instructions

Add tap water to a large shallow bowl, dip rice papers, but not for too long.

Place a large skillet over medium heat, add sesame oil.

Add tofu, soy sauce to the pan and cook for about 5 minutes until browned.

Add sesame seeds and cook for 60 seconds.

Mix the peanut dipping sauce ingredients in a bowl and set aside.

Fill rice papers with vegetables and tofu. Wrap them like a burrito.

Serve rolls with a side of peanut dipping sauce.

# 161. Turmeric Chickpea Salad Sandwich

Cooking Time: 5 minutes

Servings: 1

Ingredients

1 can chickpeas, drained

1/3 cup aquafaba : liquid from the chickpea can)

½ teaspoon turmeric

½ teaspoon onion powder

1 clove garlic, minced

salt and black pepper

Instructions

Put all ingredients into a food processor and pulse until the consistency is chunky and not smooth.

Put in a bowl and serve.

## 162. Mexican Quinoa

Cooking Time: 25 minutes

Servings: 4

Ingredients

1 cup quinoa, uncooked and rinsed

1 ½ cup vegetable broth

3 cups canned diced tomatoes

15 oz. can black beans, drained and rinsed

2 cups frozen corn

1 cup fresh parsley, chopped

1 onion, chopped

3 cloves of garlic, minced

2 bell peppers, chopped

1 tablespoon paprika powder

½ tablespoon cumin

2 tablespoons olive oil

2 tablespoons lime juice

2 green onions, chopped

salt and pepper

Instructions

Place a large pot over medium heat. Add olive oil.

Cook onions for 3 minutes.

Add garlic, bell peppers and cook for 5 minutes.

Add the remaining ingredients except lime juice, green onions and parsley. Cover and cook for about 20 minutes, keep checking to make sure the quinoa doesn't stick and burn.

Add lime juice, green onions and parsley.

Season the dish with salt and pepper before serving.

## 163. Potato Fritters

Cooking Time: 25 minutes

Servings: 12

Ingredients

For the vegetable potato fritters:

¾ cup red lentils, cooked

1 onion, chopped

2 cloves garlic, minced

2 potatoes, grated

1 carrot, grated

5 tablespoons all-purpose flour

½ teaspoon smoked paprika powder

1 teaspoon paprika powder

1 teaspoon majoram

salt and black pepper

For the Sriracha mayonnaise:

3 tablespoons vegan mayonnaise

1 teaspoon tomato paste

1 teaspoon garlic powder

½ teaspoon smoked paprika powder

Sriracha sauce

salt and pepper

Instructions

Add red lentils, carrot, potatoes, garlic, onion, flour, smoked paprika, regular paprika, Marjoram, salt and pepper to a large bowl.

Place a skillet over medium heat. Heat oil.

Scoop 2 tablespoons for each fritter and fry in the pan for about 4 minutes.

In a separate bowl combine Sriracha mayonnaise ingredients and set aside.

Serve fritters with salad and vegan sriracha mayonnaise.

## 164. Tempeh Reuben

Cooking Time: 40 minutes

Servings: 2

Ingredients

For the marinated Tempeh:

8 oz. package tempeh, thinly sliced in four

1/2 cup vegetable broth

1 tablespoon balsamic vinegar

1 tablespoon vegan Worcestershire sauce

1 teaspoon liquid smoke

1 teaspoon onion powder

1 teaspoon smoked paprika

1/2 teaspoon garlic powder

The remaining ingredients:

4 slices Alvarado's Sprouted Rye Seed Bread

1/2 heaping cup sauerkraut

1/4 cup vegan Russian Dressing

vegan Swiss cheese, sliced

2 tablespoons oil

1 tablespoon vegan butter

Instructions

Combine broth, balsamic vinegar, Worcestershire sauce, liquid smoke, onion powder, smoked paprika and garlic powder.

Add sliced tempeh to the marinade and set aside to marinate for 30 minutes.

Place a large skillet over medium heat, add oil.

Add marinated tempeh slices and cook for 5 minutes on each side, then add marinade and cook for 3 minutes.

Spread butter on the sprouted rye seed bread, place slices on the skillet and cook for 3 minutes on one side. Flip and add the Russian dressing.

Divide sauerkraut between two slices, add 2 slices of tempeh, and a slice of vegan Swiss cheese.

Add second slice of bread and toast for 5 minutes in the skillet until browned.

Remove from skillet and serve.

## 165. Broccoli Pesto with Pasta and Cherry Tomatoes

Cooking Time: 5 minutes

Servings: 2

Ingredients

For the broccoli pesto:

2 heaped cups broccoli florets, cooked

½ cup walnuts

3 tablespoons nutritional yeast

2 cloves of garlic

3 tablespoons olive oil

1/2 cup roughly chopped parsley

salt and black pepper

For the pasta:

9 oz. whole wheat pasta, cooked

1 cup cherry tomatoes, halved

1 cup cooked broccoli florets

Instructions

Combine pesto ingredients in a large bowl.

Serve cooked pasta with cherry tomatoes, cooked broccoli and pesto.

## 166. Korean Barbecue Tempeh Wraps

Cooking Time: 25 minutes

Servings: 4

Ingredients

For the Korean barbecue sauce:

¾ cup water

1/3 cup soy sauce

¼ cup maple syrup

¼ cup tomato paste

2 tablespoons gochujang

2 garlic cloves, minced

2 teaspoons ginger, grated

1 teaspoon sesame oil

For the Tempeh filling:

2 tablespoons vegetable oil

2-8 oz. packages tempeh, cubed

1 red bell pepper, thinly sliced

1 onion, thinly sliced

2 scallions, chopped

2 teaspoons sesame seeds

For the wraps:

4 large flour tortillas

4 large lettuce leaves

1 large avocado sliced

Instructions

Combine the Korean sauce ingredients in a bowl.

Place a large skillet over medium heat, add sauce and bring it to a simmer, lower the heat and let it simmer for 10 minutes.

Place another skillet over medium heat and add oil.

Add and cook tempeh for about 5 minutes.

Increase the heat, add bell pepper, onion and cook for 2 minutes, then lower the heat, add sauce and cook for 3 minutes. Once done, remove the from heat and set aside.

Put tortilla on a working surface, place lettuce leaves, avocado slices, and tempeh mixture on top. Wrap like a burrito to enclose the fillings inside

Do this for all tortillas before serving.

## 167. Crab Cakes

Cooking Time: 20 minutes

Servings: 8

Ingredients

2 cups cooked chickpeas

2 cans artichoke hearts in brine, drained and chopped

½ cup onion, chopped

¼ cup parsley, chopped

2 cloves garlic, minced

3 teaspoons fresh lemon juice

1 stalk celery, chopped

2 teaspoons Dijon mustard

3 tablespoons dill, chopped

1 cup panko bread crumbs

2 teaspoons vegan Worcestershire sauce

2 teaspoons fish seasoning

vegetable oil

salt and black pepper

Instructions

Place a skillet over medium heat. Add oil.

Sauté onions for about 2 minutes in the skillet.

Add garlic and cook 60 seconds. Remove from the heat and set aside.

Place cooked chickpeas in a bowl and mash them with a fork.

Add cooked onions, garlic and mix well.

Add the rest of the ingredients.

Season with salt and peppers. Form eight vegan crab cakes.

Place a skillet over medium heat add vegetable oil.

Add crab cakes and cook on each side for 3 minutes.

# 168. Smoky Black Beans Parsley Chimichurri

Cooking Time: 28 minutes

Servings: 3

Ingredients

For the smoky black beans:

2 teaspoons oil

15 oz. black beans

¼ cup onion, chopped

¼ cup bell pepper, chopped

2 cloves garlic, minced

½ teaspoon cumin powder

½ teaspoon chipotle chili pepper powder

½ teaspoon smoked paprika

1 medium tomato, chopped

½ zucchini, chopped

Other fillings:

Chimichurri

tortillas

2 cups baby spinach

2 red bell pepper, thinly sliced

Instructions

Place a large skillet over medium heat. Add oil.

Add and cook onions, garlic and bell peppers for about 8 minutes.

Add cumin, chili, smoked paprika, black beans, zucchini, tomato and salt. Mix, cover and cook on low medium for 10 minutes.

Place a large pan over medium heat and warm tortilla and spread Chimichurri on the tortilla.

Add black beans on the tortilla, cheese and sprinkle both bell peppers and spinach.

Wrap the tortilla before serving.

## 169. Tuna Sandwich With Chickpeas

Cooking Time: 10 minutes

Servings: 2

Ingredients

For the vegan tuna salad:

1 can chickpeas

1 tablespoon dried Wakame seaweed

2 tablespoons vegan mayonnaise

1 teaspoon soy sauce

1 teaspoon lemon juice

2 teaspoons dill

2 stalks of celery, chopped

salt and pepper

For the sandwich:

4 slices of whole wheat bread

1 tomato, thinly sliced

¼ cucumber, thinly sliced

lettuce

½ onion, cut into rings

Instructions

Crumble the weed and place in a shallow bowl.

Add water and let the weed soak for 5 minutes. Drain excess water

Place chickpeas in a large bowl and mash it with a fork.

To the bowl, add celery, mayonnaise, dill, seaweed, lemon juice, soy sauce, salt and pepper and mix well.

## 170. Sweet Potato Toast

Cooking Time: 10 minutes

Servings: 1

Ingredients

1 medium sweet potato, washed and sliced to fit into the toaster

For the chickpea topping:

1 avocado

2 cups can chickpeas, drained and rinsed

½ teaspoon sumac

1 tablespoon lemon juice

½ cup small baby watercress

For the cashew cream pepper topping:

1/3 cup cashew cream

1 pepper, thinly sliced

1 handful baby basil leaves

cracked pepper to taste

olive oil to drizzle

Instructions

Place sweet potato slices in a toaster and toast on high. Then remove from the toaster and poke. Return slices to the toaster and toast again.

Combine avocado, sumac, chickpeas, salt and lemon juice in a bowl. Mash it all together.

When sweet potatoes are well toasted, transfer them to a plate.

Spoon the chickpea mixture and spread it on sweet potato slices.

Sprinkle baby watercress and smear cashew cream on top.

Follow with basil leaves, olive oil and cracked pepper.

# 171. Chickpeas with Dates, Turmeric, Cinnamon and Almonds

Cooking Time: 2 hours

Servings: 4

Ingredients

1 2/3 cups plum tomatoes

3 1/2 oz. dates, pitted and halved

3 1/3 cups chickpeas, rinsed and drained

1.4 oz. flaked almonds, toasted

2 tablespoons olive oil

4 cloves garlic, chopped

1 tablespoon ginger, grated

1 handful coriander, stalks and leaves separated and chopped

1 teaspoon ground cumin

1 teaspoon ground coriander

1 teaspoon ground turmeric

1 cinnamon stick

1 tablespoon lemon juice

1 teaspoon lime zest

1 orange, cut into wedges

couscous to serve

Instructions

Preheat the slow cooker on low heat.

Combine 1 cup tomatoes and half of dates in a blender and blend for about 1 minute.

Add this mixture to the slow cooker with the remaining tomatoes.

To the slow cooker add oil, garlic, ginger, coriander stalks, spices, lemon zest and 1 cup water. Cook for 6 hours on low until sauce is thick.

Add chickpeas and the remaining dates and cook for ½ an hour.

Lastly add lemon juice. Remove from the slow cooker.

## 172. Cucumber Avocado Toast

Cooking time: 5 minutes

Servings: 2

Ingredients

1 cucumber, sliced

2 bread slices, toasted

¼ handful basil leaves, chopped

4 tablespoons avocado, mashed

Salt and pepper, to taste

1 teaspoon lemon juice

Instructions

1-Combine lemon juice together with the mashed avocado, and then spread the mixture on two bread slices.

2 -Top with cucumber slices along with the finely chopped basil leaves.

3-Generously sprinkle with salt and pepper and enjoy!

# 173. Tofu Fish Sticks

Cooking time: 45 minutes

Servings: 4

Ingredients

1 cup bread crumbs

2 tablespoons nori seaweed, crumbled

2 blocks tofu, pressed

2 tablespoons soy sauce

1 teaspoon lemon pepper

1/4 cup soy milk

2 tablespoons lemon juice

Directions:

Preheat the oven to 375F and then cut the tofu into strips. Evenly coat the tofu strips with flour.

Whisk the soy milk together with soy sauce and lemon juice in a bowl, and then mix the lemon pepper, breadcrumbs and nori in a separate bowl.

When done, dip the tofu in the soy milk mixture and then coat the dipped tofu in the breadcrumb's mixture.

Bake for 40-45 minutes flipping only once, until crispy and brown. Alternatively, you can fry the both sides in the pan with little oil.

When baked through, serve and enjoy!

## 174. Cornmeal Breaded Tofu

Cooking time: 15 minutes

Servings: 4

Ingredients

1/4 cup cornmeal

1/4 teaspoon cayenne pepper

1 block tofu, pressed

1 teaspoon chili powder

2 tablespoons nutritional yeast

Salt and pepper, to taste

1/4 cup flour

Olive oil

Directions:

Preheat the oven to 400F and use a kitchen brush to lightly coat the baking sheet with oil.

Cut the pressed tofu into thin rectangular strips. Mix flour, nutritionist yeast, spices and cornmeal in a bowl until well combined.

Add the tofu pieces bit by bit into the cornmeal mixture to coat evenly, and then place the coated tofu pieces on a prepared baking sheet.

Bake for 5-7 minutes until lightly browned on one side. Flip the tofu and bake for 5 more minutes until baked through. Serve.

## 175. Baked Sweet Potato Fries

Cooking time: 30 minutes

Servings: 6

Ingredients

1 tablespoon olive oil

3 large sweet potatoes, washed, peeled, chopped

1/4 teaspoon paprika

cooking spray

1 teaspoon cumin

½ teaspoon cayenne pepper

1/2 teaspoon salt

Directions:

Preheat the oven to 400F and prepare the sweet potatoes by washing and peeling them, and then chop the potatoes into wedges lengthwise.

Put the sweet potatoes wedges into a bowl and then generously drizzle them with oil and toss well until combined.

In a bowl, combine the paprika with salt and cumin, and then mix the ingredients together.

Sprinkle the cumin-paprika mixture on the sweet potato wedges and then toss well to combine, until the potatoes wedges are nicely coated with spices and olive oil.

Spray the baking sheet with cooking spray and then spread the coated sweet potatoes wedges in one layer on the sheet.

Bake the potatoes in the oven for 30 minutes.

When baked through, serve the sweet potatoes fries with your desired sauce and enjoy!

## 176. Wheat Thins

Cooking time: 15 minutes

Servings: 8

Ingredients

3 oz. water

2 1/2 oz. sugar

1/2 teaspoon ground turmeric

1 oz. coconut oil

1/2 teaspoon tartar cream

5 oz. flour

¾ oz. wheat germ, toasted

1 1/2 oz. bread flour

1/4 teaspoon baking soda

1/4 oz. barley malt syrup

1/2 teaspoon salt

Directions:

Prepare the crackers. Preheat the oven to 350F and prepare two parchment sheets. Add the sugar, wheat germ, flour, turmeric, tartar cream, coconut oil, bread flour and baking soda to a food processor bowl and blend until combined.

Add the barley malt syrup to a glass bowl along with water to dissolve the syrup, and then add into the dry blended mixture and continue processing until stiff dough is formed.

Knead the dough lightly on the surface, and then separate the dough into two equal parts.

Put the cut parchment sheets on a working surface and sprinkle with flour, and then place one of the dough halves in the middle of the paper. Sprinkle the dough with flour and roll out into the rectangle.

Use a pizza cutter cut the dough into bite-size squares and then place the crackers on a sheet pan.

Sprinkle the crackers with salt and bake for about 12 minutes. Rotate the pan halfway.

Let the crackers cool to a room temperature. When done, serve and enjoy!

# 177. Spinach and Artichoke Dip

Cooking time: 40 minutes

Servings: 6-8

Ingredients

2 tablespoons nutritional yeast

2 tablespoons olive oil

1 tablespoon Dijon mustard

1 lb. cauliflower, cored, chopped into florets

1 tablespoon lemon juice

1/4 cup vegan mayonnaise

10 oz. spinach

14 oz. artichokes drained, halved

2 oz. raw cashews

2 teaspoons garlic powder

1 cup vegetable stock or vegetable broth

2 garlic cloves, minced

Salt and pepper, to taste

Tortilla chips or pita chips, to serve

Directions:

Preheat the oven to 350F and add the vegetable stock to a skillet. Bring the vegetable stock to a simmer over medium heat and then add the cauliflower florets along with cashews and stir well until evenly coated. Set the heat to low and then close the lid. Cook for about 10 minutes until cauliflower florets are tender.

When done, transfer the cashews, cauliflower and the liquid to a blender and let cool for a minute. Process the mixture until smooth, and then add the nutritional yeast, mayonnaise, lemon juice, mustard and garlic powder, and continue processing until combined.

Use a kitchen towel to wipe the skillet and then add oil and heat on medium heat until warmed through. Add garlic and cook for 1-2 minutes until softened and fragrant, stirring frequently, and then add spinach along with salt. Continue cooking until the spinach wilts.

Add the cooked spinach to the blender along with the artichokes, and blend until incorporated.

Transfer the dip to a baking dish and bake for 30 minutes until the edges are slightly browned. Flip and bake the other side for about 2-3 minutes until nicely browned.

When baked through, serve immediately with chips and enjoy!

## 178. Coconut Bacon

Cooking time: 15 minutes

Servings: 6

Ingredients

1 teaspoon apple cider vinegar

2 tablespoons soy sauce or tamari

2 cups plain coconut flakes

2 tablespoons maple syrup

Pepper, to taste

1/2 teaspoon smoked paprika

Instructions

Preheat the oven to 325F and then add the coconut flakes to a mixing bowl.

Add all other ingredients to a separate bowl and then add the coconut flakes. Mix the ingredients together until the coconut flakes are evenly coated.

Spread the coated coconut flakes in one layer evenly on a baking sheet and bake for about 10 minutes. Stir and flip the coconut flakes, bake for 3-4 more minutes until nicely browned.

When baked through, remove from heat and let cool completely. Slice and serve.

## 179. Sweet and Sour Tofu

Preparation Time: 10 Minutes

Cooking Time: 10 Minutes

Servings: 2

Ingredients

1 cup tofu

Sea salt and pepper

½ tablespoon olive oil

1 teaspoon garlic minced

1 inch fresh ginger minced

1 large red bell pepper cut into 1-2" pieces

1/8 teaspoon red pepper flakes

1 cup vegetable stock

1/4 cup  ketchup

4 teaspoons  reduced sodium soy sauce

1 teaspoon maple syrup

½ tablespoon tapioca starch

Sliced green onions for garnish

Toasted sesame seeds for garnish

Directions:

Cut the tofu into 2-3 inch chunks. Heat up your Instant pot: press Sauté -> click on the Adjust button -> select More to get the Sauté More function, which means that the food will be sautéed over medium-high heat. Wait for the Instant Pot indicator to read HOT.

Add the olive oil to the hot Instant Pot, wait one minute for the oil to heat up and add the tofu. Sauté for 2-3 minutes, stirring a few times. Cook until it just starts to get golden.

Add the rest of the Ingredients to the Instant pot: ginger, garlic, red pepper flakes, ketchup, soy sauce, maple syrup, and stir to combine.

Add chopped bell pepper.

Close lid, select High Pressure and cook for 5 minutes.

Use a 10 minute Natural Release. Turn off the heat. Release the remaining pressure. Open the lid.

Select again the Sauté function. In a small bowl combine the tapioca starch with the vegetable stock, whisk until all combined with no lumps. Add the mixture to the Instant Pot and gently stir to combine. Cook on Sauté function for 5 more minutes, stirring occasionally, until the sauce thickens. This way you can make the sauce thicker. You can add more if you want to make the sauce even thicker, please note that it thickens as it cools too.

Turn off the Instant Pot and let the Sweet and Sour tofu stand for 5-7 minutes, the sauce will thicken more.

Serve with fresh chopped green onions, red pepper flakes and sesame seeds. Enjoy!

Nutrition:

Calories230, Total Fat 12.6g, Saturated Fat 2.1g , Cholesterol 0mg, Sodium 1110mg, Total Carbohydrate 20.9g, Dietary Fiber 2.4g , Total Sugars 13.2g , Protein 12.8g

# 180. Broccoli Tikka Masala

Preparation Time: 10 Minutes

Cooking Time: 10 Minutes

Servings: 2

Ingredients

½ tablespoon coconut oil

1 small onion, diced

1 teaspoon garlic powder

½ teaspoon ginger powder

1 teaspoon dried fenugreek leaves

1 teaspoon Garam masala

½ teaspoon turmeric

¼ teaspoon ground chili

1/8 teaspoon ground cumin

¼ teaspoon salt

2 diced tomatoes with their juice

½ tablespoon honey

1 small broccoli head, cut into florets

1/2 cup coconut cream

Directions:

Set the Instant Pot to sauté mode for 7 minutes. Add the coconut oil. Once hot, add the onion, garlic powder, and ginger powder. Cook for 3-4 minutes, or until the onions start to caramelize and become soft. Add the dried fenugreek leaves, Garam masala, turmeric, chili, cumin, and salt. Continue to cook for another 2 minutes, stirring regularly to make sure it doesn't burn. Add a couple of tablespoons of water and scrape the bottom to make sure nothing is sticking to it.

Add the diced tomatoes, honey, and broccoli florets. Secure the lid and close the vent to Sealing. Press the Pressure Cook button and adjust the time to 2 minutes. The Instant Pot will take about 10 minutes to come to pressure, then cook under pressure for 2 minutes.

Once the program is finished and you have heard the beeps, wait 1 minute and release the pressure. Stir in the coconut cream and stir to combine.

Serve hot with rice

Nutrition:

Calories 230, Total Fat 18.1g, Saturated Fat 15.7g, Cholesterol 0mg , Sodium 55mg, Total Carbohydrate 16.6g, Dietary Fiber 6.2g, Total Sugars 7.1g, Protein 5.2g

# 181. Kale with Sweet Potatoes

Preparation Time: 10 Minutes

Cooking Time: 15 Minutes

Servings: 2

Ingredients

2 cups kale washed and chopped

2 sweet potatoes washed and cut large pieces

1 cup water

1 tablespoon coconut oil

1 lime juiced, plus extra slices for serving

1tablespoon garlic powder

¼ teaspoon salt

1/8 teaspoon pepper

Directions:

Wash the kale well and chop. Wash and chop the sweet potatoes.

Add everything to the Instant Pot and stir very well.

Cover the Instant Pot and lock it in. Make sure the vent is set to "sealing".

Use the manual or pressure cook feature and set the timer for 15 minutes.

Once the timer reaches zero, quick release the pressure.

Enjoy!

Nutrition:

Calories 176, Total Fat 6.8g, Saturated Fat 5.9g, Cholesterol 0mg , Sodium 347mg, Total Carbohydrate 28.5g, Dietary Fiber 3.6g, Total Sugars 4.9g, Protein 3.8g

## 182. Steamed Vegetables

Preparation Time: 10 Minutes

Cooking Time: 10 Minutes

Servings: 2

Ingredients

3/4 cup water

½ head broccoli, chopped

½ head cauliflower, chopped

1 zucchini, chopped

½ red pepper, chopped

½ yellow pepper, chopped

¼ teaspoon salt

1/8 teaspoon pepper

Directions:

Add the 3/4 cup of water to the bottom of Instant Pot and then place trivet inside the inner pot. Add veggies, then place lid on Instant Pot and make sure valve is set to seal.

Press the pressure cook button and set to high, then cook for 0 minutes. Yes, zero minutes is all that's needed to steam! The Instant Pot will take about 5-10 minutes to come to pressure, then notify you it's done by beeping.

Press the Cancel button then do a quick release of the pressure on the Instant Pot by flicking the switch at the top with a spoon. Open the lid when pressure gauge has dropped and the lid opens easily.

Season veggies if desired then serve and enjoy!

Nutrition:

Calories62, Total Fat 0.5g, Saturated Fat 0.1g, Cholesterol 0mg , Sodium 42mg, Total Carbohydrate 13.5g, Dietary Fiber 4.2g , Total Sugars 5.2g, Protein 3.9g

# 183. Red Thai Curry Broccoli

Preparation Time: 10 Minutes

Cooking Time: 02 Minutes

Servings: 2

Ingredients

1 cup coconut milk

½ cup water

1 tablespoon red curry paste

1 teaspoon garlic minced

½ teaspoon salt plus more as needed

¼ teaspoon ginger powder

1 tablespoon onions

1/8 teaspoon chili powder

½ bell pepper any colour, thinly sliced

2 cups broccoli cut into bite-size pieces

2 cups diced tomatoes and liquid

Freshly ground black pepper

Directions:

In your Instant Pot, stir together the coconut milk, water, red curry paste, minced garlic, salt, ginger powder, onion, and chili powder. Add the bell pepper, broccoli, and tomatoes, and stir again. Lock the lid and turn the steam release handle to Sealing. Using the Manual or Pressure Cook function, set the cooker to High Pressure for 2 minutes./

When the cook time is complete, quick release the pressure.

Carefully remove the lid and give the whole thing a good stir. Taste and season with more salt and pepper, as needed. Serve with rice

Nutrition:

Calories 190, Total Fat 4.8g, Saturated Fat 1g, Cholesterol 0mg , Sodium 987mg, Total Carbohydrate 29.9g, Dietary Fiber 7.9g, Total Sugars 15.4g, Protein 9.2g

## 184. Lime Ginger Green Beans

Preparation Time: 05 Minutes

Cooking Time: 0 Minutes

Servings: 2

Ingredients

2 cups green beans cut into 4 inches

1 cup water

1 tablespoon vegetable oil

2 teaspoons freshly squeezed lime juice

½ teaspoon salt

1 teaspoon ginger powder

Directions:

Place the green beans in a steamer basket and put the basket into the Instant Pot. Add the water. Lock the lid and turn the steam release handle to Sealing. Using the Manual or Pressure Cook function, set the cooker to Low Pressure for 0 minutes.

When the cook time is complete, quick release the pressure.

In a serving bowl, stir together the vegetable oil, lime juice, salt, and ginger powder.

Carefully remove the lid and add the green beans to the bowl. Toss to combine. Taste and add the remaining lemon juice and/or ginger, as needed.

Nutrition:

Calories108, Total Fat 7g, Saturated Fat 1.4g, Cholesterol 0mg , Sodium 593mg, Total Carbohydrate 12.2g, Dietary Fiber 4.1g, Total Sugars 2.3g, Protein 2.3g

## 185. Kale Tofu Curry

Preparation Time: 05 Minutes

Cooking Time: 20 Minutes

Servings: 2

Ingredients

1-1/2 tablespoons coconut oil

¼ onion finely chopped

½ green chili finely chopped

½ tablespoon Ginger-Garlic paste

2 cups kale

1/2 cup water

1 cup tofu cubes

2 tablespoons coconut cream to garnish

1 medium tomato finely chopped

½ tablespoon cumin seeds

1 tablespoon coriander powder

1 teaspoon Garam masala powder

Red chili powder to taste

Salt to taste

Directions:

Put instant pot on sauté high mode. Add coconut oil and let it get hot, add cumin seeds and fry well.

Add onions and green chili, sauté, then add tomatoes, fry till mushy.

Add in the spice powders and salt, mix well, then add in the kale, water and mix. Turn off sauté mode.

Put the lid, vent to sealing position. Do manual high 2 minutes and Quick release after 2 minutes in warm mode.

Now grind the kale onion tomato mix using a hand blender or in a regular blender to a fine paste. Add in more water to desired consistency and put on sauté mode high for 5 minutes or so.

Add Garam masala and mix, then add in the tofu cubes and simmer for 2 to 4 minutes.

Serve with coconut cream if desired.

Nutrition:

Calories 254, Total Fat 13.7g, Saturated Fat 9g, Cholesterol 0mg, Sodium 131mg, Total Carbohydrate 30.2g, Dietary Fiber 2.2g , Total Sugars 12.1g, Protein 5.5g

# 186. Potato and Broccoli Curry

Preparation Time: 10 Minutes

Cooking Time: 10 Minutes

Servings: 2

Ingredients

1 tablespoon avocado oil

1 teaspoon mustard seed

1 onion chopped

½ tablespoon hot curry powder

1 cup ripe tomatoes

2 potatoes unpeeled and cut

Salt and pepper

1 medium broccoli cut into large : 3-inchflorets, stalk and core discarded

Directions:

Put the avocado oil in the Instant pot, select SAUTÉ, and adjust to NORMAL/MEDIUM heat. When the oil is hot, add the mustard seeds and cook until they have popped and turned grey, 1 minute. Add the onions and curry powder and cook, stirring frequently, until the onions are tender, 4 minutes. Add the tomatoes and cook until they break down a bit, about 2 minutes. Press CANCEL.

Add the potatoes, 1/2 cup water, 1 teaspoon salt, and several grinds of pepper and stir into the tomato mixture. Place the broccoli florets on top of the potato mixture, but don't stir. Lock on the lid, select the PRESSURE COOK function, and adjust to LOW pressure for 2 minutes. Make sure the steam valve is in the "Sealing" position.

When the cooking time is up, quick-release the pressure. Pour the mixture into a large serving bowl and break up the broccoli a bit with a spoon. Serve immediately.

Nutrition:

Calories 206, Total Fat 2.4g, Saturated Fat 0.3g, Cholesterol 0mg , Sodium 122mg, Total Carbohydrate 44.3g, Dietary Fiber 7.1g , Total Sugars 6.8g, Protein 6.9g

## 187. Turnips in Cilantro Gravy

Preparation Time: 10 Minutes

Cooking Time: 15 Minutes

Servings: 2

Ingredients

7 turnips

¼ tablespoon cumin seeds

¼ tablespoon mustard seeds

1 tablespoon coconut oil

1/4 cup water

½ bunch fresh cilantro

Green chilies to taste

Salt to taste

½ teaspoon ginger powder

1 tablespoon tamarind pulp

Directions:

Grind cilantro, green chilli, salt, ginger powder and tamarind pulp using little or no water. Wash the turnips and make crisps cross slits till 3/4th length of turnips.

Stuff the ground cilantro paste into the turnips along the slits. Keep aside. Now put instant pot sauté mode high, add coconut oil.

Once the oil is hot add cumin seeds and mustard seeds, fry well. Turn off sauté mode.

Add the stuffed turnips in one layer, then add the remaining cilantro paste. Add little water 1/4 cup to 1/2 cup.

Mix gently : optional). Put the lid and vent to sealing position.

Do manual "low pressure" 5 minutes. Quick release after 2 minutes in warm mode.

The eggplants should be cooked by now. Serve with Rice.

Nutrition:

Calories202, Total Fat 7.5g, Saturated Fat 5.9g, Cholesterol 0mg , Sodium 363mg, Total Carbohydrate 31.7g, Dietary Fiber 7.7g , Total Sugars 19.9g, Protein 4.3g

## 188. Bell Peppers & Sweet Potato Stir Fry

Preparation Time: 05 Minutes

Cooking Time: 15 Minutes

Servings: 2

Ingredients

½ tablespoon avocado oil

1 bell pepper cut in long pieces

2 sweet potatoes, cut into small pieces.

¼ teaspoon cumin seeds

1 teaspoon garlic powder

¼ tablespoon lemon juice

Basil to garnish

1/8 teaspoon turmeric powder

¼ teaspoon red chili powder

½ teaspoon coriander powder

½ teaspoon salt

Directions:

Heat instant pot in sauté mode and add avocado oil in it. Add cumin and garlic powder.

Once the cumin and garlic powder turns golden brown, add the cut bell peppers, sweet potatoes and turmeric powder, coriander powder, red chilli powder and salt. Mix well. Sprinkle water with your hand.

Change the instant pot setting to manual mode or pressure cook mode, at high pressure for 2 minutes. Keep the vent in sealed position.

When the instant pot beeps, quick release the pressure manually. The veggies would be cooked. If they are watery, change the instant pot setting to sauté mode and stir until you get the desired consistency.

Stir in the lemon juice and mix well.

Garnish with fresh basil and enjoy.

Nutrition:

Calories209, Total Fat 1g, Saturated Fat 0.2g, Cholesterol 0mg , Sodium 601mg, Total Carbohydrate 48.1g, Dietary Fiber 7.5g , Total Sugars 4.2g, Protein 3.4g

## 189. Cauliflower Stir-Fry

Preparation Time: 10 Minutes

Cooking Time: 05 Minutes

Servings: 2

Ingredients

½ tablespoon coconut oil

1 small onion, sliced thin

½ cup diagonally sliced zucchini

1 cup cauliflower florets

1 cup green peas

½ large red bell pepper, cut into strips

½ tablespoon reduced sodium soy sauce

1 teaspoon minced garlic

1 teaspoon ginger, crushed

1 teaspoon sesame Seed, toasted

Directions:

Heat instant pot in sauté mode and add coconut oil in it. Add onion and minced garlic and crushed ginger.

Once the onion turns golden brown, add the cut bell peppers, zucchini, cauliflower, green peas. Mix well. Sprinkle water and soy sauce with your hand.

Change the instant pot setting to manual mode or pressure cook mode, at high pressure for 2 minutes. Keep the vent in sealed position.

When the instant pot beeps, quick release the pressure manually. The veggies would be cooked. If they are watery, change the instant pot setting to sauté mode and stir until you get the desired consistency.

Garnish with sesame seed and enjoy.

Nutrition:

Calories145, Total Fat 4.7g, Saturated Fat 3.1g, Cholesterol 0mg , Sodium 174mg, Total Carbohydrate 21.4g, Dietary Fiber 6.8g , Total Sugars 8.9g, Protein 6.6g

# 190. Easy Sweet Potato Asparagus

Preparation Time: 05Minutes

Cooking Time: 10 Minutes

Servings: 2

Ingredients

½ tablespoon coconut oil

¼ teaspoon cumin seeds

½ teaspoon garlic powder

1 green chili chopped

1 cup asparagus chopped in 1/2 inch pieces

½ sweet potato cubed into small pieces

1 teaspoon coriander powder

1/8 teaspoon turmeric powder

1/8 teaspoon red chili powder

½ teaspoon salt

½ teaspoon dry mango

Directions:

Start the Instant Pot in Sauté mode, heat it and then add coconut oil. Heating the pot first helps later, so the veggies don't stick to the bottom. Then add cumin seeds, garlic powder and green chili.

When the cumin seeds start to splutter, add chopped asparagus and sweet potatoes. Add turmeric powder, red chilli powder, coriander powder and salt and mix properly. Sprinkle water with your hand.

Close the instant pot lid, and change setting to manual mode for 2 minutes. When the instant pot beeps, let the pressure release naturally.

Mix in the dry mango powder. If there is any water, change the setting to sauté mode and get it to your desired consistency.

Served with roti.

Nutrition:

Calories 98, Total Fat 3.7g, Saturated Fat 3g, Cholesterol 0mg, Sodium 597mg, Total Carbohydrate 16.3g, Dietary Fiber 3.5g , Total Sugars 4.2g, Protein 2.3g

# 191. Ginger Veggie Stir-Fry

Preparation Time: 05Minutes

Cooking Time: 10 Minutes

Servings: 2

Ingredients

½ tablespoon corn-starch

2 teaspoons garlic powder

2 teaspoons ginger powder

1/4 cup olive oil, divided

1 small head broccoli, cut into florets

1/2 cup snow peas

3/4 cup julienned carrots

1/2 cup halved green beans

2 tablespoons soy sauce

2 1/2 tablespoons water

1/4 cup chopped onion

½ tablespoon salt

Directions:

In a large bowl, blend corn-starch, garlic, 1 teaspoon ginger, and 2 tablespoons vegetable oil until corn-starch is dissolved. Mix in broccoli, snow peas, carrots, and green beans, tossing to lightly coat.

Start the Instant Pot in Sauté mode, heat it and then add coconut oil. Put all vegetable in the pot and sauté for 2 minutes then add soy sauce and water . Mix well.

Close the instant pot lid, and change setting to manual mode for 5 minutes. When the instant pot beeps, let the pressure release naturally.

If there is any water, change the setting to sauté mode and get it to your desired consistency.

Serve.

Nutrition:

Calories304, Total Fat 25.6g, Saturated Fat 3.7g, Cholesterol 0mg , Sodium 2693mg, Total Carbohydrate 18g, Dietary Fiber 4.3g , Total Sugars 6g, Protein 4.7g

## 192. Cottage cheese and Potato Coconut Curry

Preparation Time: 10 Minutes

Cooking Time: 10 Minutes

Servings: 2

Ingredients

1 package cottage cheese

1 cup vegetable broth

1 cup onion sliced

¼ teaspoon Ginger powder

1/8 teaspoon turmeric powder

½ teaspoon cumin

1 cup potatoes diced

1 cup coconut milk unsweetened

Salt to taste

Pepper to taste

Directions:

In an Instant Pot, heat about 1/4 cup of the vegetable broth on medium to high heat.

Add onions, ginger, turmeric and cumin and sauté. Add potatoes and sauté a few minutes.

Crumble cottage cheese into tiny pieces : resembling ground meat), mix well, and then add coconut milk.

Close the Instant Pot and Cook at low pressure for 4 minutes by using the Manual setting, adjusting pressure to low, and setting cook time to 4 minutes.

When time is up, use a quick release.

Remove the lid and, uncovered, simmer until liquid is absorbed. Add salt and pepper

Nutrition:

Calories233, Total Fat 5.2g, Saturated Fat 3.6g, Cholesterol 9mg , Sodium 930mg, Total Carbohydrate 26.4g, Dietary Fiber 3g , Total Sugars 3.7g, Protein 20.4g

# 193. Rutabagas Curry

Preparation Time: 10 Minutes

Cooking Time: 20 Minutes

Servings: 2

Ingredients

4 rutabagas peeled and cored from the top

1 tablespoon vegetable oil

½ onion finely chopped

1 teaspoon ginger powder

1 teaspoon garlic powder

1 red tomato pureed

¼ teaspoon turmeric

¼ tablespoon red chili powder

¼ teaspoon Garam masala

½ teaspoon salt

5 almonds

1/8 cup milk warm

½ tablespoon dried fenugreek leaves

Basil leaves

Directions:

Soak almonds in warm milk for 10 minutes and set aside.

Set Instant Pot to sauté mode. Once the 'hot' sign displays, add vegetable oil. Add onions and cook for 2 minutes with a glass lid on, stirring few times.

Add ginger and garlic powder, cook for 30 seconds. Add the carved out pieces from the rutabagas.

Add tomato paste, turmeric, red chili powder, Garam masala and salt. Cook everything on sauté mode for 2 minutes with glass lid on, stirring a couple of times.

With a small spoon, very carefully fill the rutabagas with the cooked masala/gravy and line them all in the Instant Pot insert.

Add 1/2 cup of water. Close the Instant Pot, set on Manual at high pressure for 8 minutes. When time is up, quick release the pressure

Blend milk and almonds together to make smooth paste.

Stir in dried fenugreek leaves, almond paste and chopped basil.

Set Instant Pot to sauté mode, mix everything together. Add salt to taste. Bring to gentle boil and then turn Instant Pot off.

Serve with hot and. Enjoy!

Nutrition:

Calories219, Total Fat 9.4g, Saturated Fat 1.7g, Cholesterol 1mg , Sodium 664mg, Total Carbohydrate 31g, Dietary Fiber 9.3g, Total Sugars 18.7g, Protein 6.2g

## 194. Spice-Rubbed Broccoli Steaks

Preparation Time: 10 Minutes

Cooking Time: 05 Minutes

Servings: 2

Ingredients

1 small head broccoli

1 tablespoon coconut oil

1 teaspoon red chilli powder

1 teaspoon ground cumin

½ teaspoon salt

½ cup parsley fresh, chopped

½ lemon

Directions:

Insert the steam rack into the Instant Pot. Add 1 1/2 cups water

Remove the leaves from the broccoli and trim the core so the broccoli sits flat. Place on the steam rack.

In a small bowl, combine the coconut oil, red chilli powder, cumin, and salt. Drizzle over the broccoli and rub to coat.

Lock the lid. Press [Manual] and cook on high pressure for 4 minutes. Use the "Quick Release" method to vent the steam, then open the lid.

Lift the broccoli onto a cutting board and slice into 1-inch-thick steaks. Divide among plates and sprinkle with the parsley.

Serve with the lemon quarters. Enjoy!

Nutrition:

Calories 78, Total Fat 7g, Saturated Fat 5.9g, Cholesterol 0mg , Sodium 597mg, Total Carbohydrate 4.4g, Dietary Fiber 1.6g , Total Sugars 1.1g, Protein 1.4g

# 195. Spicy Eggplant

Preparation Time: 10 Minutes

Cooking Time: 20 Minutes

Servings: 2

Ingredients

1 tablespoon coconut oil

2 eggplants, cut into 1-inch cubes

1 onion, thinly sliced

½ tablespoon garlic powder

1 tablespoon soy sauce

1 cup water

1 teaspoon honey

 Ground black pepper to taste

Salt to taste

Directions:

Set Instant Pot to sauté mode, heat coconut oil. Cook and stir the eggplant cubes until they begin to brown, 3 to 5 minutes. Remove the eggplant with a slotted spoon, and set aside.

Then add onions just until they begin to soften, about 30 seconds. Stir in the garlic powder, and cook and stir an additional 30 seconds. Mix in the soy sauce, water, honey, and black pepper, and stir to form a smooth sauce. Return the eggplant to the Instant pot, Lock the lid. Press [Manual] and cook on high pressure for 5 minutes. Use the "Quick Release" method to vent the steam, then open the lid.

Serve.

Nutrition:

Calories240, Total Fat 7.9g, Saturated Fat 5.9g , Cholesterol 0mg, Sodium 546mg, Total Carbohydrate 42.4g, Dietary Fiber 20.8g , Total Sugars 22.3g, Protein 6.9g

# 196. Cottage Chesses Peanut Stir-Fry

Preparation Time: 10 Minutes

Cooking Time: 10 Minutes

Servings: 2

Ingredients

2 tablespoons vegetable oil

½ cup frozen stir-fry vegetables

¼ teaspoon ginger powder

Salt and pepper to taste

1 egg, beaten

¼ cup corn-starch

1 cup cottage cheese, drained and cubed

1/8 cup peanut sauce

1 tablespoon chopped peanuts

Directions:

Turn Instant Pot to Sauté mode. Once the "hot" sign displays add the vegetable oil and add vegetables until tender. Mix in the ginger powder, and season with salt and pepper. Remove vegetables from pot, and set aside.

Place the egg in a bowl. In a separate bowl, mix the corn-starch, salt, and pepper. Dip cottage cheese cubes first in the egg, then the corn-starch mixture to coat.

Heat the remaining oil in the Instant pot to Sauté mode, and cook the coated cottage cheese 5 minutes, or until golden brown. Stir in the peanut sauce and peanuts. Continue to cook and stir until sauce has thickened and cottage cheese is well-coated. Serve with the vegetables.

Nutrition:

Calories394, Total Fat 25.5g, Saturated Fat 5.8g, Cholesterol 91mg , Sodium 899mg, Total Carbohydrate 17.4g, Dietary Fiber 2.2g , Total Sugars 8.9g, Protein 22.8g

## 197. Tofu Teriyaki

Preparation Time: 05 Minutes

Cooking Time: 15 Minutes

Servings: 2

Ingredients

½ cup vegetable broth

1/8 cup tamari sauce

1/8 cup onion peeled and chopped

½ tablespoon honey

½ tablespoon ginger powder

¼ tablespoon garlic powder

1 cup tofu cubed

Directions:

Mix the broth, tamari, onion, honey, ginger powder, and garlic powder in an Instant Pot. Add the tofu, stir well, and lock the lid to the Instant pot.

Press Pressure cook on Max pressure for 10 minutes with the Keep Warm setting off.

When the machine has finished cooking, turn it off and let its pressure return to normal naturally, about 25 minutes. Unlatch the lid and open the cooker. Use tongs or a slotted spoon to transfer the tofu to a bowl.

Press the button for SAUTE. Set it for HIGH, MORE or CUSTOM 400°F. Set the time for 15 minutes and if necessary, press START.

Bring the sauce in the pot to a boil, stirring often. Continue boiling, stirring more and more frequently until almost constantly, until the sauce is a thick glaze, about 7 minutes. Turn off the SAUTÉ function. Return the tofu and any juices to the cooker. Stir until the tofu coated in the glaze. Transfer the pieces to a serving platter or plates.

Nutrition:

Calories136, Total Fat 5.7g, Saturated Fat 1.2g, Cholesterol 0mg , Sodium 1213mg, Total Carbohydrate 10.1g, Dietary Fiber 1.7g, Total Sugars 6.2g, Protein 13.8g

# 198. Zesty Lemon Jackfruit

Preparation Time: 05 Minutes

Cooking Time: 20 Minutes

Servings: 2

Ingredients

½ teaspoon red chilli powder

¼ teaspoon salt

¼ pepper

1 cup jackfruit

2 tablespoons coconut oil

1/2 small onion chopped

1 teaspoon garlic powder

½ teaspoon dried basil lightly crushed

1/8 cup lemon juice

Zest of one lemon

1 tablespoon chopped fresh coriander

Lemon slices for garnish

Directions:

Mix red chilli powder, salt and pepper in a small bowl. Coat tops : smooth sideof tofu in seasoning mixture.

Add coconut oil to the Instant Pot. Using the display panel select the SAUTE function.

When oil gets hot, brown the jackfruit on both sides, 3-4 minutes per side. Do not crowd the pot--you may have to work in batches. Transfer browned jackfruit to a shallow dish and cover loosely with foil.

Add onion and remaining oil to the Instant pot and sauté until soft, 3-4 minutes. Add garlic powder and crushed basil and cook for 1-2 minutes more.

Add lemon juice and zest to the Instant pot and deglaze by using a wooden spoon to scrape the brown bits from the bottom of the pot.

Put the jackfruit back into to the Instant pot in one even layer, seasoned side up.

Turn the pot off by selecting CANCEL, then secure the lid, making sure the vent is closed.

Using the display panel select the MANUAL or PRESSURE COOK function*. Use the + /- keys and program the Instant Pot for 7 minutes.

When the time is up, let the pressure naturally release for 5 minutes, then quick-release the remaining pressure.

Serve jackfruit topped with fresh coriander and lemon slices.

Nutrition:

Calories 207, Total Fat 13.9g, Saturated Fat 11.8g, Cholesterol 0mg , Sodium 295mg, Total Carbohydrate 23g , Dietary Fiber 2.2g, Total Sugars 1.1g, Protein 1.6g

# 199. Coconut Potato Curry

Preparation Time: 05 Minutes

Cooking Time: 10 Minutes

Servings: 2

Ingredients

Coconut potato Curry:

½ tablespoon coconut oil

1 cup potatoes cubes

1 small onion finely diced

1 teaspoon garlic powder

½ teaspoon ginger powder

1 cup coconut milk full fat

Spice Mixture:

½ tablespoon curry powder

½ tablespoon dried rosemary

½ teaspoon salt

¼ teaspoon chili powder

1/8 teaspoon pepper

¼ teaspoon cardamom

To Finish:

1tablespoon corn-starch

1/8 cup chopped cilantro for garnish

Directions:

Add coconut oil to the Instant Pot. Using the display panel select the SAUTE function.

When oil gets hot, brown the potatoes on both sides, 2-3 minutes per side. Add onion, garlic powder and ginger powder to the pot and sauté 2 minutes. Stir in the Spice Mixture Ingredients and cook for 1 minute more.

Add coconut milk to the Instant pot and deglaze by using a wooden spoon to scrape the brown bits from the bottom of the pot.

Turn the Instant pot off by selecting CANCEL, then secure the lid, making sure the vent is closed.

Using the display panel select the MANUAL or PRESSURE COOK function. Use the + /- keys and program the Instant Pot for 5 minutes.

When the time is up, quick-release the pressure.

Carefully remove 1/4 cup of the liquid from the Instant pot and combine with the corn-starch. Stir into the Instant pot until thickened. Serve with cilantro

Nutrition:

Calories 400, Total Fat 32.6g, Saturated Fat 28.5g, Cholesterol 0mg, Sodium 615mg, Total Carbohydrate 28.3g, Dietary Fiber 5.8g , Total Sugars 6.5g, Protein 5.5g

## 200. Herb and Garlic Cottage Cheese

Preparation Time: 35 Minutes

Cooking Time: 20 Minutes

Servings: 2

Ingredients

1 tablespoon coconut oil

½ tablespoon prepared Dijon Mustard

½ tablespoon apple cider vinegar

1 teaspoon Garlic powder

½ teaspoon pepper

¼ teaspoon salt

2 cups cottage cheese

1 tablespoon butter

1 teaspoon garlic powder

1/4 cup water

1/8 cup cream

½ tablespoon corn-starch

Directions:

In a medium bowl, whisk together the marinade coconut oil, Dijon mustard, apple cider vinegar, garlic powder, pepper, salt. Add the cottage cheese and allow it to marinate for 30 minutes.

Add coconut oil to the Instant Pot. Using the display panel select the SAUTE function. When the coconut oil is melted, add garlic powder to the Instant pot and sauté 2-3 minutes.

Drain the cottage cheese, but reserve the marinade. Brown the cottage cheese on both sides, 3-4 minutes per side.

Add reserved marinade and 1/4 cup water to the pot and deglaze by using a wooden spoon to scrape the brown bits from the bottom of the pot.

Put the cottage cheese back into to the Instant  pot, turning once to coat.

Turn the Instant pot off by selecting CANCEL, then secure the lid, making sure the vent is closed.

Using the display panel select the MANUAL or PRESSURE COOK function. Use the + /- keys and program the Instant Pot for 5 minutes.

When the time is up, let the pressure naturally release for 10 minutes, then quick-release the remaining pressure.

In a small bowl, mix together cream and corn-starch. Stir into the Instant pot until thickened, returning to SAUTE mode as needed.

Serve cottage cheese topped with sauce.

Nutrition:

Calories 333, Total Fat 17.8g, Saturated Fat 12.8g, Cholesterol 36mg , Sodium 1346mg, Total Carbohydrate 10.1g, Dietary Fiber 0.3g , Total Sugars 1.4g, Protein 31.5g

## 201. Cilantro Lime Eggplant with avocado

Preparation Time: 05 Minutes

Cooking Time: 20 Minutes

Servings: 2

Ingredients

1-1/2 cups fresh salsa

½ tablespoon taco seasoning

Zest and juice of 1 lime

¼ cup Water

2 eggplants

1 jalapeno seeded and diced : optional

½ cup chopped fresh cilantro

Avocado

Directions:

Add all Ingredients to the Instant pot and stir to combine.

Secure the lid, making sure the vent is closed.

Using the display panel select the MANUAL or PRESSURE COOK function. Use the + /- keys and program the Instant Pot for 12 minutes.

When the time is up, let the pressure naturally release for 10 minutes, then quick-release the remaining pressure.

Add cilantro. Stir to combine.

 Garnish with lime wedges and cheese.

Nutrition:

Calories534Total Fat 31.3g, Saturated Fat 7.5g, Cholesterol 23mg , Sodium 1049mg, Total Carbohydrate 56.9g, Dietary Fiber 28.2g , Total Sugars 18.6g, Protein 17.7g

## 202. Peanut Chutney Mushrooms with Tamarind

Preparation Time: 15 Minutes

Cooking Time: 15 Minutes

Servings: 2

Ingredients

1-1/2 tablespoons olive oil divided

½ cup raw peanuts

1 dried red Chile

½ tablespoon cumin seeds

½ tablespoon coriander seeds

5 curry leaves torn into pieces

½ teaspoon kosher salt divided

1 tablespoon tamarind concentrate

Water

2 onions diced

½ teaspoon ginger powder

½ teaspoon garlic powder

1 cup mushrooms cut into 1 inch pieces

Directions:

Using the Sauté function on high, heat 1 tablespoon oil in the Instant pot for about 1 minute, until shimmering. Add the peanuts and cook for 1 minute, stirring frequently, until fragrant. Add the chilies, cumin seeds, coriander seeds and curry leaves; cook for 1 minute, until fragrant. Transfer the nuts and spices to a blender and let cool slightly. Remove 1/4 cup of the peanut mixture and set aside. Add 1 teaspoon salt and the tamarind concentrate to the blender; blend on high speed until smooth, adding 1 tablespoon water if needed to help the mixture blend.

Using the Sauté function on high, heat 2 tablespoons oil in the Instant pot for about 1 minute, until shimmering. Add the onions and cook for about 4 minutes, stirring occasionally, until softened. Add the ginger and garlic; cook for about 1 minute, until fragrant.

Stir in the mushrooms, 1/2 cup water, peanut chutney and remaining 1 teaspoon salt. Secure the lid and cook on high pressure for 8 minutes.

Once the cooking is complete, let the pressure release naturally for 10 minutes, then quick-release the remaining pressure. Transfer the curry to a platter. Pour the reserved peanuts and spices over the mushrooms and serve.

Nutrition:

Calories353, Total Fat 26.3g, Saturated Fat 3.6g, Cholesterol 0mg , Sodium 605mg, Total Carbohydrate 24.1g, Dietary Fiber 8g, Total Sugars 9.2g, Protein 12.9g

## 203.Tofu with 20 Cloves of Garlic

Preparation Time: 05 Minutes

Cooking Time: 15 Minutes

Servings: 2

Ingredients

2 cups tofu cut into pieces

1/4 teaspoon sea salt

½ tablespoon coconut oil

20 cloves garlic or more

½ teaspoon basil chopped

½ teaspoon rosemary chopped

½ teaspoon thyme chopped

½ cup vegetable stock

1 tablespoon coconut cream

1 tablespoon arrowroot

Directions:

Season the pieces of tofu with sea salt.

Select the sauté setting on your Instant pot, allowing it to come up to temperature.

Add ¼   tablespoon of coconut oil to the instant pot, and swirl around.

Add half of the tofu pieces, and sear on the other side for 4 minutes. Set this tofu aside, and repeat with the remaining tofu.

Add the garlic cloves to the Instant pot, and sauté for 1-2 minutes, stirring frequently.

Turn off the sauté setting.

Add the tofu back into the Instant Pot and sprinkle it liberally with the chopped herbs.

Add the vegetable stock to the Instant pot, then seal the lid.

Select high, and time for 10 minutes.

Once the timer has gone off, allow the Instant Pot to gradually depressurize about 10 minutes. Remove the tofu and set aside to keep warm.

Turn the sauté function back on high.

Add the coconut cream to the Instant pot with the stock and garlic and stir gently.

Dilute the arrowroot in some water and stir in gradually to thicken the sauce.

After it has thickened to a rich consistency, pour the creamy garlic clove sauce over the tofu and serve.

Nutrition:

Calories 272, Total Fat 15.9g, Saturated Fat 6.7g, Cholesterol 0mg , Sodium 284mg, Total Carbohydrate 15.4g, Dietary Fiber 3.3g , Total Sugars 2.2g, Protein 23g

# 204. Mushrooms and Olive Curry

Preparation Time: 15 Minutes

Cooking Time: 15 Minutes

Servings: 2

Ingredients

1 teaspoon red chilli powder

½ teaspoon ground cumin

½ teaspoon turmeric powder

¼ teaspoon ground ginger

1/8 teaspoon ground cinnamon

2 cups mushrooms

Salt and pepper

2 tablespoons vegetable oil

1 onion sliced

1 teaspoon garlic powder

1 tablespoon tomato paste

1 cup vegetable broth

¼ lemon juiced

¼ cup  high-quality pitted olives

Directions:

Combine the red chilli powder, cumin, turmeric, ginger powder, and cinnamon in a small bowl. season the mushrooms generously with salt and pepper on it. place in a bowl or plastic bag to marinate for at least 1 hour.

Once the mushrooms is done marinating, turn on the sauté function of Instant pot. once hot, add the vegetable oil. add mushrooms, and cook for about 3 minutes without moving. set aside.

Add the onion and cook for 2 minutes, scraping the bottom of the Instant pot. add the garlic powder and tomato paste and cook, stirring, for 1 more minute. turn off the sauté function. add the broth and scrape any remaining bits off the bottom of the Instant pot. add the mushrooms, and squeeze them in so that they fit in one layer. secure the lid.

Cook at high pressure for 05 minutes and use a natural release.

Remove the mushrooms and some of the onions. turn on the sauté function and simmer the sauce for 10 to 15 minutes, until reduced by more than half and starting to thicken. turn off the sauté function. add the lemon juice, stir, and taste for seasoning.

To serve, pour the sauce over the mushrooms and sprinkle the olives on top.

Nutrition:

Calories199, Total Fat 16.8g, Saturated Fat 3.2g, Cholesterol 0mg , Sodium 555mg, Total Carbohydrate 9.3g, Dietary Fiber 2.8g , Total Sugars 3.5g, Protein 5.8g

## 205. Apricot Tempeh

Preparation Time: 15 Minutes

Cooking Time: 10 Minutes

Servings: 2

Ingredients

2 cups tempeh

¼ teaspoon salt

1/8 teaspoon black pepper

½ tablespoon olive oil

1 small onion chopped

½ cup vegetable broth divided

½ teaspoon ginger powder

½ teaspoon garlic powder

¼ teaspoon ground cinnamon

1/16 teaspoon ground allspice

2 cups diced tomatoes

4 ounces dried apricots

Basil chopped fresh

Directions:

Season both sides of tempeh with 1/4 teaspoon salt and 1/8 teaspoon pepper. Press Sauté; heat oil in Instant Pot. Add tempeh, cook about 8 minutes or until browned on both sides. Remove to plate.

Add onion and 2 tablespoons broth to Instant pot; cook and stir 5 minutes or until onion is translucent, scraping up browned bits from bottom of pot.

Add ginger powder, garlic powder, cinnamon and allspice; cook and stir 30 seconds or until fragrant.

Stir in tomatoes, apricots, remaining broth and saffron, if desired; mix well. Return tempeh to pot, pressing into liquid.

Secure lid and move pressure release valve to sealing position. Press Manual; cook at high pressure 5 minutes.

When cooking is complete, press Cancel and use quick release. Season with additional salt and pepper.

Garnish with basil and serve.

Nutrition:

Calories 439, Total Fat 22.6g, Saturated Fat 4.4g, Cholesterol 0mg, Sodium 508mg, Total Carbohydrate 33.6g, Dietary Fiber 4.4g , Total Sugars 11.7g, Protein 35g

# Chapter 6. Vegetables

## 206. Simple Carrots Mix

Preparation time: 10 minutes

Cooking time: 40 minutes

Servings: 6

Ingredients:

15 carrots, halved lengthwise

2 tablespoons coconut sugar

¼ cup olive oil

½ teaspoon rosemary, dried

½ teaspoon garlic powder

A pinch of black pepper

Directions:

In a bowl, combine the carrots with the sugar, oil, rosemary, garlic powder and black pepper, toss well, spread on a lined baking sheet, introduce in the oven and bake at 400 degrees F for 40 minutes.

Divide between plates and serve as a side dish.

Enjoy!

Nutrition: calories 211, fat 2, fiber 6, carbs 14, protein 8

## 207. Tasty Grilled Asparagus

Preparation time: 10 minutes

Cooking time: 6 minutes

Servings: 4

Ingredients:

2 pounds asparagus, trimmed

2 tablespoons olive oil

A pinch of salt and black pepper

Directions:

In a bowl, combine the asparagus with salt, pepper and oil and toss well.

Place the asparagus on preheated grill over medium-high heat, cook for 3 minutes on each side, divide between plates and serve as a side dish.

Enjoy!

Nutrition: calories 172, fat 4, fiber 7, carbs 14, protein 8

## 208. Easy Roasted Carrots

Preparation time: 10 minutes

Cooking time: 30 minutes

Servings: 4

Ingredients:

2 pounds carrots, quartered

A pinch of black pepper

3 tablespoons olive oil

2 tablespoons parsley, chopped

Directions:

Arrange the carrots on a lined baking sheet, add black pepper and oil, toss, introduce in the oven and cook at 400 degrees F for 30 minutes.

Add parsley, toss, divide between plates and serve as a side dish.

Enjoy!

Nutrition: calories 177, fat 3, fiber 6, carbs 14, protein 6

## 209. Oven Roasted Asparagus

Preparation time: 10 minutes

Cooking time: 25 minutes

Servings: 4

Ingredients:

2 pounds asparagus spears, trimmed

3 tablespoons olive oil

A pinch of black pepper

2 teaspoons sweet paprika

1 teaspoon sesame seeds

Directions:

Arrange the asparagus on a lined baking sheet, add oil, black pepper and paprika, toss, introduce in the oven and bake at 400 degrees F for 25 minutes.

Divide the asparagus between plates, sprinkle sesame seeds on top and serve as a side dish.

Enjoy!

Nutrition: calories 190, fat 4, fiber 8, carbs 11, protein 5

## 210. Baked Potato Mix

Preparation time: 10 minutes

Cooking time: 1 hour and 15 minutes

Servings: 8

Ingredients:

6 potatoes, peeled and sliced

2 garlic cloves, minced

2 tablespoons olive oil

1 and ½ cups coconut cream

¼ cup coconut milk

1 tablespoon thyme, chopped

¼ teaspoon nutmeg, ground

A pinch of red pepper flakes

1 and ½ cups low-fat cheddar, shredded

½ cup low-fat parmesan, grated

Directions:

Heat up a pan with the oil over medium heat, add garlic, stir and cook for 1 minute.

Add coconut cream, coconut milk, thyme, nutmeg and pepper flakes, stir, bring to a simmer, reduce heat to low and cook for 10 minutes.

Arrange 1/3 of the potatoes in a baking dish, add 1/3 of the cream, repeat with the rest of the potatoes and the cream, sprinkle the cheddar on top, cover with tin foil, introduce in the oven and cook at 375 degrees F for 45 minutes.

Uncover the dish, sprinkle the parmesan, bake everything for 20 minutes, divide between plates and serve as a side dish.

Enjoy!

Nutrition: calories 224, fat 8, fiber 9, carbs 16, protein 15

## 211. Spicy Brussels Sprouts

Preparation time: 10 minutes

Cooking time: 20 minutes

Servings: 6

Ingredients:

2 pounds Brussels sprouts, halved

2 tablespoons olive oil

A pinch of black pepper

1 tablespoon sesame oil

2 garlic cloves, minced

½ cup coconut aminos

2 teaspoons apple cider vinegar

1 tablespoon coconut sugar

2 teaspoons chili sauce

A pinch of red pepper flakes

Sesame seeds for serving

Directions:

Spread the sprouts on a lined baking dish, add the olive oil, the sesame oil, black pepper, garlic, aminos, vinegar, coconut sugar, chili sauce and pepper flakes, toss well, introduce in the oven and bake at 425 degrees F for 20 minutes.

Divide the sprouts between plates, sprinkle sesame seeds on top and serve as a side dish.

Enjoy!

Nutrition: calories 176, fat 3, fiber 6, carbs 14, protein 9

## 212. Baked Cauliflower

Preparation time: 10 minutes

Cooking time: 30 minutes

Servings: 4

Ingredients:

3 tablespoons olive oil

2 tablespoons chili sauce

Juice of 1 lime

3 garlic cloves, minced

1 cauliflower head, florets separated

A pinch of black pepper

1 teaspoon cilantro, chopped

Directions:

In a bowl, combine the oil with the chili sauce, lime juice, garlic and black pepper and whisk.

Add cauliflower florets, toss, spread on a lined baking sheet, introduce in the oven and bake at 425 degrees F for 30 minutes.

Divide the cauliflower between plates, sprinkle cilantro on top and serve as a side dish.

Enjoy!

Nutrition: calories 188, fat 4, fiber 7, carbs 14, protein 8

## 213. Baked Broccoli

Preparation time: 10 minutes

Cooking time: 15 minutes

Servings: 4

Ingredients:

1 tablespoon olive oil

1 broccoli head, florets separated

2 garlic cloves, minced

½ cup coconut cream

½ cup low-fat mozzarella, shredded

¼ cup low-fat parmesan, grated

A pinch of pepper flakes, crushed

Directions:

In a baking dish, combine the broccoli with oil, garlic, cream, pepper flakes and mozzarella and toss.

Sprinkle the parmesan on top, introduce in the oven and bake at 375 degrees F for 15 minutes.

Divide between plates and serve as a side dish.

Enjoy!

Nutrition: calories 188, fat 4, fiber 7, carbs 14, protein 7

## 214. Easy Slow Cooked Potatoes

Preparation time: 10 minutes

Cooking time: 6 hours

Servings: 6

Ingredients:

Cooking spray

2 pounds baby potatoes, quartered

3 cups low-fat cheddar cheese, shredded

2 garlic cloves, minced

8 bacon slices, cooked and chopped

¼ cup green onions, chopped

1 tablespoon sweet paprika

A pinch of black pepper

Directions:

Spray a slow cooker with the cooking spray, add baby potatoes, cheddar, garlic, bacon, green onions, paprika and black pepper, toss, cover and cook on High for 6 hours.

Divide between plates and serve as a side dish.

Enjoy!

Nutrition: calories 200, fat 4, fiber 6, carbs 12, protein 7

## 215. Mashed Potatoes

Preparation time: 10 minutes

Cooking time: 20 minutes

Servings: 6

Ingredients:

3 pounds potatoes, peeled and cubed

2 tablespoons non-fat butter

½ cup coconut milk

A pinch of salt and black pepper

½ cup low-fat sour cream

Directions:

Put the potatoes in a pot, add water to cover, add a pinch of salt and pepper, bring to a boil over medium heat, cook for 20 minutes and drain.

Add butter, milk and sour cream, mash well, stir everything, divide between plates and serve as a side dish.

Enjoy!

Nutrition: calories 188, fat 3, fiber 7, carbs 14, protein 8

## 216. Squash Side Salad

Preparation time: 10 minutes

Cooking time: 30 minutes

Servings: 6

Ingredients:

1 cup orange juice

3 tablespoons coconut sugar

1 and ½ tablespoons mustard

1 tablespoon ginger, grated

1 and ½ pounds butternut squash, peeled and roughly cubed

Cooking spray

A pinch of black pepper

1/3 cup olive oil

6 cups salad greens

1 radicchio, sliced

½ cup pistachios, roasted

Directions:

In a bowl, combine the orange juice with the sugar, mustard, ginger, black pepper and squash, toss well, spread on a lined baking sheet, spray everything with cooking oil, introduce in the oven and bake at 400 degrees F for 30 minutes.

In a salad bowl, combine the squash with salad greens, radicchio, pistachios and oil, toss well, divide between plates and serve as a side dish.

Enjoy!

Nutrition: calories 275, fat 3, fiber 4, carbs 16, protein 6

## 217. Colored Iceberg Salad

Preparation time: 10 minutes

Cooking time: 0 minutes

Servings: 4

Ingredients:

1 iceberg lettuce head, leaves torn

6 bacon slices, cooked and halved

2 green onions, sliced

3 carrots, shredded

6 radishes, sliced

¼ cup red vinegar

¼ cup olive oil

3 garlic cloves, minced

A pinch of black pepper

Directions:

In a large salad bowl, combine the lettuce leaves with the bacon, green onions, carrots, radishes, vinegar, oil, garlic and black pepper, toss, divide between plates and serve as a side dish.

Enjoy!

Nutrition: calories 235, fat 4, fiber 4, carbs 10, protein 6

## 218. Fennel Side Salad

Preparation time: 10 minutes

Cooking time: 0 minutes

Servings: 4

Ingredients:

2 fennel bulbs, trimmed and shaved

1 and ¼ cups zucchini, sliced

2/3 cup dill, chopped

¼ cup lemon juice

¼ cup olive oil

6 cups arugula

½ cups walnuts, chopped

1/3 cup low-fat feta cheese, crumbled

Directions:

In a large bowl, combine the fennel with the zucchini, dill, lemon juice, arugula, oil, walnuts and cheese, toss, divide between plates and serve as a side dish.

Enjoy!

Nutrition: calories 188, fat 4, fiber 5, carbs 14, protein 6

# 219. Corn Mix

Preparation time: 10 minutes

Cooking time: 0 minutes

Servings: 4

Ingredients:

½ cup cider vinegar

¼ cup coconut sugar

A pinch of black pepper

4 cups corn

½ cup red onion, chopped

½ cup cucumber, sliced

½ cup red bell pepper, chopped

½ cup cherry tomatoes, halved

3 tablespoons parsley, chopped

1 tablespoon basil, chopped

1 tablespoon jalapeno, chopped

2 cups baby arugula leaves

Directions:

In a large bowl, combine the corn with onion, cucumber, bell pepper, cherry tomatoes, parsley, basil, jalapeno and arugula and toss.

Add vinegar, sugar and black pepper, toss well, divide between plates and serve as a side dish.

Enjoy!

Nutrition: calories 100, fat 2, fiber 3, carbs 14, protein 4

## 220. Persimmon Side Salad

Preparation time: 10 minutes

Cooking time: 0 minutes

Servings: 4

Ingredients:

Seeds from 1 pomegranate

2 persimmons, cored and sliced

5 cups baby arugula

6 tablespoons green onions, chopped

4 navel oranges, peeled and cut into segments

¼ cup white vinegar

1/3 cup olive oil

3 tablespoons pine nuts

1 and ½ teaspoons orange zest, grated

2 tablespoons orange juice

1 tablespoon coconut sugar

½ shallot, chopped

A pinch of cinnamon powder

Directions:

In a salad bowl, combine the pomegranate seeds with persimmons, arugula, green onions and oranges and toss.

In another bowl, combine the vinegar with the oil, pine nuts, orange zest, orange juice, sugar, shallot and cinnamon, whisk well, add to the salad, toss and serve as a side dish.

Enjoy!

Nutrition: calories 188, fat 4, fiber 4, carbs 14, protein 4

## 221. Avocado Side Salad

Preparation time: 10 minutes

Cooking time: 0 minutes

Servings: 4

Ingredients:

4 blood oranges, peeled and cut into segments

2 tablespoons olive oil

A pinch of red pepper, crushed

2 avocados, peeled, pitted and cut into wedges

1 and ½ cups baby arugula

¼ cup almonds, toasted and chopped

1 tablespoon lemon juice

Directions:

In a bowl, combine the oranges with the oil, red pepper, avocados, arugula, almonds and lemon juice, toss, divide between plates and serve as a side dish.

Enjoy!

Nutrition: calories 231, fat 4, fiber 8, carbs 16, protein 6

## 222. Classic Side Dish Salad

Preparation time: 10 minutes

Cooking time: 0 minutes

Servings: 4

Ingredients:

3 garlic cloves, minced

Juice of ½ lemon

6 ounces coconut cream

2 lettuce hearts, torn

1 cup corn

4 ounces green beans, halved

1 cup cherry tomatoes, halved

1 cucumber, chopped

1/3 cup chives, chopped

1 avocado, peeled, pitted and halved

6 bacon slices, cooked and chopped

Directions:

In a bowl, combine the lettuce with corn, green beans, cherry tomatoes, cucumber, chives, avocado and bacon and toss.

In another bowl, combine the garlic with lemon juice and coconut cream, whisk well, add to the salad, toss and serve as a side dish.

Enjoy!

Nutrition: calories 175, fat 12, fiber 4, carbs 13, protein 6

## 223. Easy Kale Mix

Preparation time: 10 minutes

Cooking time: 0 minutes

Servings: 4

Ingredients:

1 whole wheat bread slice, toasted and torn into small pieces

6 tablespoons low-fat cheddar, grated

3 tablespoons olive oil

5 tablespoons lemon juice

1 garlic clove, minced

7 cups kale, torn

A pinch of black pepper

Directions:

In a bowl, combine the bread with cheese and kale.

In another bowl, combine the oil with the lemon juice, garlic and black pepper, whisk, add to the salad, toss, divide between plates and serve as a side dish.

Enjoy!

Nutrition: calories 200, fat 4, fiber 5, carbs 14, protein 8

## 224. Asparagus Salad

Preparation time: 10 minutes

Cooking time: 4 minutes

Servings: 4

Ingredients:

4 tablespoons avocado oil

2 tablespoons balsamic vinegar

1 tablespoon coconut aminos

1 garlic clove, minced

1 pound asparagus, trimmed

6 cups frisee lettuce leaves, torn

1 cup edamame, shelled

1 cup parsley, chopped

Directions:

Heat up a pan with 1 tablespoon oil over medium-high heat, add asparagus, cook for 4 minutes and transfer to a salad bowl.

Add lettuce, edammae and parsley and toss.

In another bowl, combine the rest of the oil with the vinegar, aminos and garlic, whisk well, add over the salad, toss, divide between plates and serve as a side dish.

Enjoy!

Nutrition: calories 200, fat 4, fiber 5, carbs 14, protein 6

## 225. Green Side Salad

Preparation time: 10 minutes

Cooking time: 0 minutes

Servings: 4

Ingredients:

4 cups baby spinach leaves

1 cucumber, sliced

3 ounces broccoli florets

3 ounces green beans, blanched and halved

¾ cup edamame, shelled

1 and ½ cups green grapes, halved

1 cup orange juice

¼ cup olive oil

1 tablespoon cider vinegar

2 tablespoons parsley, chopped

2 teaspoons mustard

A pinch of black pepper

Directions:

In a salad bowl, combine the baby spinach with cucumber, broccoli, green beans, edamame and grapes and toss.

Add orange juice, olive oil, vinegar, parsley, mustard and black pepper, toss well, divide between plates and serve as a side dish.

Enjoy!

Nutrition: calories 117, fat 4, fiber 5, carbs 14, protein 4

# 226. Baked Zucchini

Preparation time: 10 minutes

Cooking time: 20 minutes

Servings: 4

Ingredients:

4 zucchinis, quartered lengthwise

½ teaspoon thyme, dried

½ teaspoon oregano, dried

½ cup low-fat parmesan, grated

½ teaspoon basil, dried

¼ teaspoon garlic powder

2 tablespoons olive oil

2 tablespoons parsley, chopped

A pinch of black pepper

Directions:

Arrange zucchini pieces on a lined baking sheet, add thyme, oregano, basil, garlic powder, oil, parsley and black pepper and toss well.

Sprinkle parmesan on top, introduce in the oven and bake at 350 degrees F for 20 minutes.

Divide between plates and serve as a side dish.

Enjoy!

Nutrition: calories 198, fat 4, fiber 4, carbs 14, protein 5

## 227. Baked Mushrooms

Preparation time: 10 minutes

Cooking time: 15 minutes

Servings: 4

Ingredients:

1 and ½ pounds white mushrooms, sliced

¼ cup lemon juice

3 tablespoons olive oil

Zest of 1 lemon, grated

3 garlic cloves, minced

2 teaspoons thyme, dried

¼ cup low-fat parmesan, grated

A pinch of salt and black pepper

Directions:

In a bowl, combine the mushrooms with the lemon juice, oil, lemon zest, garlic, thyme, parmesan, salt and pepper, toss, spread on a lined baking sheet, introduce in the oven at 375 degrees F for 15 minutes, divide between plates and serve as a side dish.

Enjoy!

Nutrition: calories 164, fat 12, fiber 3, carbs 10, protein 7

## 228. Garlic Potatoes

Preparation time: 10 minutes

Cooking time: 30 minutes

Servings: 6

Ingredients:

3 pounds red potatoes, halved

4 garlic cloves, minced

2 tablespoons olive oil

1 teaspoon thyme, dried

½ teaspoon basil, dried

1/3 cup low-fat parmesan, grated

2 tablespoons low-fat butter, melted

2 tablespoons parsley, chopped

Black pepper to the taste

Directions:

In a roasting pan, combine the red potatoes with garlic, oil, thyme, basil, parmesan, butter and black pepper, toss, introduce in the oven and cook at 400 degrees F for 30 minutes.

Add parsley, toss, divide between plates and serve as a side dish.

Enjoy!

Nutrition: calories 251, fat 12, fiber 4, carbs 13, protein 6

## 229. Corn Pudding

Preparation time: 10 minutes

Cooking time: 15 minutes

Servings: 4

Ingredients:

8 ears corn, grated

3 bacon slices, chopped

1 yellow onion, chopped

½ cup coconut milk

½ cup basil, torn

A pinch of black pepper

½ teaspoon red pepper flakes

Directions:

Heat up a pan over medium-high heat, add bacon, stir and cook for 2 minutes.

Add corn, onion, black pepper and pepper flakes, stir and cook for 8 minutes.

Add milk and basil, stir and cook for 5 minutes more, divide between plates and serve as a side dish.

Enjoy!

Nutrition: calories 201, fat 3, fiber 5, carbs 14, protein 7

## 230. Corn Sauté

Preparation time: 10 minutes

Cooking time: 12 minutes

Servings: 4

Ingredients:

4 cups corn

4 bacon slices, cut into strips

A pinch of red pepper flakes

3 scallions, chopped

A pinch of black pepper

Directions:

Heat up a pan over medium-high heat, add bacon, toss and cook for 5 minutes.

Add corn, pepper flakes, black pepper and scallions, toss, cook for 7 minutes more, divide between plates and serve as a side dish.

Enjoy!

Nutrition: calories 199, fat 3, fiber 6, carbs 13, protein 8

## 231. Pineapple Potato Salad

Preparation time: 10 minutes

Cooking time: 40 minutes

Servings: 4

Ingredients:

2 cups pineapple, peeled and cubed

4 sweet potatoes, cubed

1 tablespoon olive oil

¼ cup coconut, unsweetened and shredded

1/3 cup almonds, chopped

1 cup coconut cream

Directions:

Arrange sweet potatoes on a lined baking sheet, add the olive oil, introduce in the oven at 350 degrees F, roast for 40 minutes, put them in a salad bowl, add coconut, pineapple, almonds and cream, toss, divide between plates and serve as a side dish.

Enjoy!

Nutrition: calories 200, fat 4, fiber 3, carbs 7, protein 8

## 232. Coconut Sweet Potatoes

Preparation time: 10 minutes

Cooking time: 1 hour

Servings: 4

Ingredients:

4 sweet potatoes, sliced

A drizzle of olive oil

A pinch of salt and black pepper

1 small thyme bunch, chopped

1/3 cup coconut cream

½ teaspoon parsley, chopped

1 tablespoon Dijon mustard

½ teaspoon garlic

Directions:

Arrange sweet potato slices on a lined baking sheet, sprinkle thyme, drizzle oil, season with a pinch of salt and black pepper, toss well, introduce in the oven at 400 degrees F and bake for about 1 hour.

Meanwhile, in a bowl, mix coconut cream with parsley, garlic and mustard and whisk well.

Arrange baked potatoes on plates, drizzle the mustard sauce all over and serve as a side dish.

Enjoy!

Nutrition: calories 237, fat 5, fiber 4, carbs 12, protein 9

## 233. Cashew And Coconut Sweet Potatoes

Preparation time: 10 minutes

Cooking time: 1 hour

Servings: 4

Ingredients:

2 sweet potatoes, peeled and sliced

½ cup cashews, soaked for a couple of hours and drained

1 cup coconut milk

¼ teaspoon cinnamon powder

Directions:

In your food processor, mix cashews, milk and cinnamon and pulse.

Spread some of the potato slices in a greased baking pan and drizzle some of the cashews cream.

Repeat with the rest of the potatoes and cream, bake in the oven for 1 hour at 350 degrees F, divide between plates and serve as a side dish.

Enjoy!

Nutrition: calories 200, fat 5, fiber 3, carbs 9, protein 8

## 234. Sage Celery Mix

Preparation time: 10 minutes

Cooking time: 10 minutes

Servings: 6

Ingredients:

2 tablespoons olive oil

5 celery ribs, chopped

1 yellow onion, chopped

1 teaspoon sage, dried

8 ounces walnuts, chopped

A pinch of black pepper

3 tablespoons sage, chopped

Directions:

Heat up a pan with the oil over medium heat, add celery and onion, stir and cook for 5 minutes.

Add dried sage, pepper, fresh sage and walnuts, stir, cook for 5 minutes more, divide between plates and serve as a side dish.

Enjoy!

Nutrition: calories 250, fat 7, fiber 5, carbs 9, protein 4

## 235. Garlic Zucchini Fries

Preparation time: 10 minutes

Cooking time: 20 minutes

Servings: 4

Ingredients:

4 zucchinis, cut into medium fries

A pinch of black pepper

½ teaspoon chili powder

1 tablespoon olive oil

¼ teaspoon garlic powder

Directions:

Spread the zucchini fries on a lined baking sheet, add black pepper, chili powder, garlic powder and oil, toss, introduce in the oven, bake at 400 degrees F for 20 minutes, divide between plates and serve as a side dish.

Enjoy!

Nutrition: calories 185, fat 3, fiber 2, carbs 6, protein 8

## 236. Tahini Green Beans

Preparation time: 10 minutes

Cooking time: 10 minutes

Servings: 4

Ingredients:

1 and ½ tablespoons tahini paste

Juice of 1 lemon

Zest of 1 lemon, grated

2 tablespoons olive oil

1 garlic clove, minced

1 red onion, sliced

1 yellow bell pepper, sliced

10 ounces green beans, halved

A pinch of black pepper

Directions:

In a bowl, mix lemon zest, lemon juice, tahini and black pepper and whisk well.

Heat up a pan with the oil over medium-high heat, add onion, stir and cook  for 5 minutes.

Add the bell pepper, garlic and green beans, toss and cook for 10 minutes.

Add tahini dressing, toss, cook for 2 minutes more, divide between plates and serve as a side dish.

Enjoy!

Nutrition: calories 180, fat 10, fiber 6, carbs 13, protein 8

## 237. Mustard Tarragon Beets

Preparation time: 10 minutes

Cooking time: 0 minutes

Servings: 5

Ingredients:

1 tablespoon Dijon mustard

1 and ½ tablespoon olive oil

8 ounces beets, cooked and sliced

2 tablespoons tarragon, chopped

A pinch of black pepper

Directions:

In a bowl, mix mustard with oil and black pepper and whisk.

In a bowl, combine the beets with the tarragon and the mustard mix, toss, divide between plates and serve as a side dish.

Enjoy!

Nutrition: calories 170, fat 5, fiber 7, carbs 8, proteins 10

## 238. Almond Green Beans

Preparation time: 10 minutes

Cooking time: 20 minutes

Servings: 6

Ingredients:

5 tablespoons olive oil

3 pounds green beans, halved

8 tablespoons almonds, toasted and sliced

A pinch of black pepper

2 yellow onions, chopped

2 and ½ tablespoons parsley, chopped

Directions:

Heat up a pan over medium-high heat, add green beans, cook them for 5 minutes and transfer to a bowl.

Heat up the same pan with the olive oil over medium heat, add onions and a pinch of black pepper, stir and cook for 10 minutes.

Add beans, almonds and parsley, toss, cook for 5 minutes, divide between plates and serve as a side dish.

Enjoy!

Nutrition: calories 130, fat 1, fiber 2, carbs 7, protein 6

## 239. Tomatoes Side Salad

Preparation time: 10 minutes

Cooking time: 0 minutes

Servings: 4

Ingredients:

½ bunch mint, chopped

8 plum tomatoes, sliced

1 teaspoon mustard

1 tablespoon rosemary vinegar

A pinch of black pepper

Directions:

In a bowl, mix vinegar with mustard and pepper and whisk.

In another bowl, combine the tomatoes with the mint and the vinaigrette, toss, divide between plates and serve as a side dish.

Enjoy!

Nutrition: calories 70, fat 2, fiber 2, carbs 6, protein 4

# 240. Squash Salsa

Preparation time: 10 minutes

Cooking time: 13 minutes

Servings: 6

Ingredients:

3 tablespoons olive oil

5 medium squash, peeled and sliced

1 cup pepitas, toasted

7 tomatillos

A pinch of black pepper

1 small onion, chopped

2 tablespoons fresh lime juice

2 tablespoons cilantro, chopped

Directions:

Heat up a pan over medium heat, add tomatillos, onion and black pepper, stir, cook for 3 minutes, transfer to your food processor and pulse.

Add lime juice and cilantro, pulse again and transfer to a bowl.

Heat up your kitchen grill over high heat, drizzle the oil over squash slices, grill them for 10 minutes, divide them between plates, add pepitas and tomatillos mix on top and serve as a side dish.

Enjoy!

Nutrition: calories 120, fat 2, fiber 1, carbs 7, protein 1

## 241. Apples And Fennel Mix

Preparation time: 10 minutes

Cooking time: 0 minutes

Servings: 3

Ingredients:

3 big apples, cored and sliced

1 and ½ cup fennel, shredded

1/3 cup coconut cream

3 tablespoons apple vinegar

½ teaspoon caraway seeds

Black pepper to the taste

Directions:

In a bowl, mix fennel with apples and toss.

In another bowl, mix coconut cream with vinegar, black pepper and caraway seeds, whisk well, add over the fennel mix, toss, divide between plates and serve as a side dish.

Enjoy!

Nutrition: calories 130, fat 3, fiber 6, carbs 10, protein 3

## 242. Simple Roasted Celery Mix

Preparation time: 10 minutes

Cooking time: 25 minutes

Servings: 3

Ingredients:

3 celery roots, cubed

2 tablespoons olive oil

A pinch of black pepper

2 cups natural and unsweetened apple juice

¼ cup parsley, chopped

¼ cup walnuts, chopped

Directions:

In a baking dish, combine the celery with the oil, pepper, parsley, walnuts and apple juice, toss to coat, introduce in the oven at 450 degrees F, bake for 25 minutes, divide between plates and serve as a side dish.

Enjoy!

Nutrition: calories 140, fat 2, fiber 2, carbs 7, protein 7

## 243. Thyme Spring Onions

Preparation time: 10 minutes

Cooking time: 40 minutes

Servings: 8

Ingredients:

15 spring onions

A pinch of black pepper

1 teaspoon thyme, chopped

1 tablespoon olive oil

Directions:

Put onions in a baking dish, add thyme, black pepper and oil, toss, bake in the oven at 350 degrees F for 40 minutes, divide between plates and serve as a side dish.

Enjoy!

Nutrition: calories 120, fat 2, fiber 2, carbs 7, protein 2

## 244. Carrot Slaw

Preparation time: 10 minutes

Cooking time: 10 minutes

Servings: 4

Ingredients:

¼ yellow onion, chopped

5 carrots, cut into thin matchsticks

1 tablespoon olive oil

1 garlic clove, minced

1 tablespoon Dijon mustard

1 tablespoon red vinegar

A pinch of black pepper

1 tablespoon lemon juice

Directions:

In a bowl, mix vinegar with black pepper, mustard and lemon juice and whisk.

Heat up a pan with the oil over medium heat, add onion, stir and cook for 5 minutes.

Add garlic and carrots, stir, cook for 5 minutes more, transfer to a salad bowl, cool down, add the vinaigrette, toss, divide between plates and serve as a side dish.

Enjoy!

Nutrition: calories 120, fat 3, fiber 3, carbs 7, protein 5

# 245. Watermelon Tomato Salsa

Preparation time: 10 minutes

Cooking time: 0 minutes

Servings: 16

Ingredients:

4 yellow tomatoes, seedless and chopped

A pinch of black pepper

1 cup watermelon, seedless and chopped

1/3 cup red onion, chopped

2 jalapeno peppers, chopped

¼ cup cilantro, chopped

3 tablespoons lime juice

Directions:

In a bowl, mix tomatoes with watermelon, onion and jalapeno.

Add cilantro, lime juice and pepper, toss, divide between plates and serve as a side dish.

Enjoy!

Nutrition: calories 87, fat 1, fiber 2, carbs 4, protein 7

## 246. Sprouts Side Salad

Preparation time: 10 minutes

Cooking time: 0 minutes

Servings: 4

Ingredients:

2 zucchinis, cut with a spiralizer

2 cups bean sprouts

4 green onions, chopped

1 red bell pepper, chopped

Juice of 1 lime

1 tablespoon olive oil

½ cup cilantro, chopped

¾ cup almonds, chopped

Black pepper to the taste

Directions:

In a salad bowl, mix zucchinis with bean sprouts, onions and bell pepper.

Add black pepper, lime juice, almonds, cilantro and olive oil, toss everything, divide between plates and serve as a side dish.

Enjoy!

Nutrition: calories 120, fat 4, fiber 2, carbs 7, protein 12

## 247. Cabbage Slaw

Preparation time: 10 minutes

Cooking time: 0 minutes

Servings: 4

Ingredients:

1 green cabbage head, shredded

1/3 cup coconut, shredded

¼ cup olive oil

2 tablespoons lemon juice

¼ cup coconut aminos

3 tablespoons sesame seeds

½ teaspoon curry powder

1/3 teaspoon turmeric powder

½ teaspoon cumin, ground

Directions:

In a bowl, mix cabbage with coconut and lemon juice and stir.

Add oil, aminos, sesame seeds, curry powder, turmeric and cumin, toss to coat and serve as a side dish.

Enjoy!

Nutrition: calories 130, fat 4, fiber 5, carbs 8, protein 6

## 248. Edamame Side Salad

Preparation time: 10 minutes

Cooking time: 0 minutes

Servings: 4

Ingredients:

1 tablespoon ginger, grated

2 green onions, chopped

3 cups edamame, blanched

2 tablespoons rice vinegar

1 tablespoon sesame seeds

Directions :

In a bowl, combine the ginger with the onions, edamame, vinegar and sesame seeds, toss, divide between plates and serve as a side dish.

Enjoy!

Nutrition: calories 120, fat 3, fiber 2, carbs 5, protein 9

## 249. Flavored Beets Side Salad

Preparation time: 10 minutes

Cooking time: 0 minutes

Servings: 4

Ingredients:

4 carrots, sliced

12 radishes, sliced

1 beet, peeled and grated

2 tablespoons raisins

Juice of 2 lemons

1 sugar beet, peeled and chopped

1 tablespoon chives, chopped

1 tablespoon parsley, chopped

1 tablespoon lemon thyme, chopped

1 tablespoon white sesame seeds

4 handfuls spinach leaves

4 tablespoons olive oil

Black pepper to the taste

Directions:

In a salad bowl, mix carrots, radishes, beets, sugar beet, raisins, chives, parsley, spinach, thyme and sesame seeds.

Add lemon juice, oil and black pepper, toss well and serve as a side dish.

Enjoy!

Nutrition: calories 110, fat 2, fiber 2, carbs 4, protein 7

## 250. Tomato And Avocado Salad

Preparation time: 10 minutes

Cooking time: 0 minutes

Servings: 4

Ingredients:

1 cucumber, chopped

1 pound tomatoes, chopped

2 avocados, pitted, peeled and chopped

1 small red onion, sliced

2 tablespoons olive oil

2 tablespoons lemon juice

¼ cup cilantro, chopped

Black pepper to the taste

Directions:

In a salad bowl, mix tomatoes with onion, avocado, cucumber and cilantro.

In a small bowl, mix oil with lemon juice and black pepper, whisk well, pour this over the salad, toss and serve as a side dish.

Enjoy!

Nutrition: calories 120, fat 2, fiber 2, carbs 3, protein 4

## 251. Greek Side Salad

Preparation time: 10 minutes

Cooking time: 0 minutes

Servings: 4

Ingredients:

4 pounds heirloom tomatoes, sliced

1 yellow bell pepper, thinly sliced

1 green bell pepper, thinly sliced

1 red onion, thinly sliced

Black pepper to the taste

½ teaspoon oregano, dried

2 tablespoons mint leaves, chopped

A drizzle of olive oil

Directions:

In a salad bowl, mix tomatoes with yellow and green peppers, onion, salt and pepper, toss to coat and leave aside for 10 minutes.

Add oregano, mint and olive oil, toss to coat and serve as a side salad.

Enjoy!

Nutrition: calories 100, fat 2, fiber 2, carbs 3, protein 6

## 252. Cucumber Salad

Preparation time: 10 minutes

Cooking time: 0 minutes

Servings: 4

Ingredients:

2 English cucumbers, chopped

8 dates, pitted and sliced

¾ cup fennel, sliced

2 tablespoons chives, chopped

½ cup walnuts, chopped

2 tablespoons lemon juice

4 tablespoons olive oil

Black pepper to the taste

Directions:

In a salad bowl, combine the cucumbers with dates, fennel, chives, walnuts, lemon juice, oil and black pepper, toss, divide between plates and serve as a side dish.

Enjoy!

Nutrition: calories 100, fat 1, fiber 1, carbs 7, protein 6

## 253. Black Beans And Veggies Side Salad

Preparation time: 10 minutes

Cooking time: 0 minutes

Servings: 4

Ingredients:

1 big cucumber, cut into chunks

15 ounces canned black beans, no-salt-added, drained and rinsed

1 cup corn

1 cup cherry tomatoes, halved

1 small red onion, chopped

3 tablespoons olive oil

4 and ½ teaspoons orange marmalade

Black pepper to the taste

½ teaspoon cumin, ground

1 tablespoon lemon juice

Directions:

In a bowl, mix beans with cucumber, corn, onion and tomatoes.

In another bowl, mix marmalade with oil, lemon juice, black pepper to the taste and cumin, whisk, pour over the salad, toss and serve as a side dish.

Enjoy!

Nutrition: calories 110, fat 0, fiber 3, carbs 6, protein 8

## 254. Endives And Escarole Side Salad

Preparation time: 10 minutes

Cooking time: 0 minutes

Servings: 4

Ingredients:

1 teaspoon shallot, minced

¼ cup apple cider vinegar

1 teaspoon Dijon mustard

3 Belgian endives, roughly chopped

¾ cup olive oil

1 cup escarole leaves, torn

Directions:

In a bowl, mix escarole leaves with endives, shallot, vinegar, mustard and oil, toss, divide between plates and serve as a side salad.

Enjoy!

Nutrition: calories 100, fat 1, fiber 3, carbs 6, protein 7

## 255. Radicchio And Lettuce Side Salad

Preparation time: 10 minutes

Cooking time: 0 minutes

Servings: 4

Ingredients:

½ cup olive oil

Black pepper to the taste

2 tablespoons shallot, chopped

¼ cup mustard

Juice of 2 lemons

½ cup basil, chopped

5 baby romaine lettuce heads, chopped

3 radicchios, sliced

3 endives, roughly chopped

Directions:

In a salad bowl, mix romaine lettuce with radicchios and endives.

In another bowl, mix oil with the pepper, shallot, mustard, lemon juice and basil, whisk, add to the salad, toss and serve as a side salad.

Enjoy!

Nutrition: calories 120, fat 2, fiber 1, carbs 8, protein 2

## 256. Jicama Side Salad

Preparation time: 10 minutes

Cooking time: 0 minutes

Servings: 4

Ingredients:

1 romaine lettuce head, leaves torn

1 Jicama, peeled and grated

1 cup cherry tomatoes, halved

1 yellow bell pepper, chopped

1 cup carrot, shredded

3 ounces low-fat cheese, crumbled

3 tablespoons red wine vinegar

5 tablespoons non-fat yogurt

1 and ½ tablespoons olive oil

1 teaspoon parsley, chopped

1 teaspoon dill, chopped

Black pepper to the taste

Directions:

In a salad bowl, mix lettuce leaves with Jicama, tomatoes, bell pepper and carrot and toss.

In another bowl, combine the cheese with vinegar, yogurt, oil, pepper, dill and parsley, whisk, add to the salad, toss to coat, divide between plates and serve as a side dish.

Enjoy!

Nutrition: calories 170, fat 4, fiber 8, carbs 14, protein 11

## 257. Cauliflower Risotto

Preparation time: 10 minutes

Cooking time: 7 minutes

Servings: 4

Ingredients:

2 tablespoons olive oil

2 garlic cloves, minced

12 ounces cauliflower rice

2 tablespoons thyme, chopped

1 tablespoon lemon juice

Zest of ½ lemon, grated

A pinch of black pepper

Directions:

Heat up a pan with the oil over medium-high heat, add cauliflower rice and garlic, stir and cook for 5 minutes.

Add lemon juice, lemon zest, thyme, salt and pepper, stir, cook for 2 minutes more, divide between plates and serve as a side dish.

Enjoy!

Nutrition: calories 130, fat 2, fiber 2, carbs 6, protein 8

## 258. Cranberry And Broccoli Mix

Preparation time: 10 minutes

Cooking time: 0 minutes

Servings: 4

Ingredients:

½ cup avocado mayonnaise

1 tablespoon apple cider vinegar

1 tablespoon lemon juice

1 tablespoon coconut sugar

¼ cup cranberries

½ cup almonds, sliced

9 ounces broccoli florets, separated

Directions:

In a bowl, mix broccoli with cranberries and almond slices and toss.

In another bowl, mix coconut sugar with vinegar, mayo and lemon juice, whisk well, add to the broccoli mix, toss, divide between plates and serve as a side dish.

Enjoy!

Nutrition: calories 120, fat 1, fiber 3, carbs 7, protein 8

## 259. Three Beans Mix

Preparation time: 10 minutes

Cooking time: 0 minutes

Servings: 4

Ingredients:

15 ounces canned kidney beans, no-salt-added, drained and rinsed

15 ounces canned garbanzo beans, no-salt-added and drained

15 ounces canned pinto beans, no-salt- added and drained

3 tablespoons balsamic vinegar

2 tablespoons olive oil

2 teaspoon Italian seasoning

2 teaspoons garlic powder

1 teaspoon onion powder

Directions:

In a large salad bowl, combine the beans with vinegar, oil, seasoning, garlic powder and onion powder, toss, divide between plates and serve as a side dish.

Enjoy!

Nutrition: calories 140, fat 1, fiber 10, carbs 10, protein 7

## 260. Creamy Cucumber Mix

Preparation time: 10 minutes

Cooking time: 0 minutes

Servings: 2

Ingredients:

1 big cucumber, peeled and chopped

1 small red onion, chopped

4 tablespoons non-fat yogurt

1 teaspoon balsamic vinegar

Directions:

In a bowl, mix onion with cucumber, yogurt and vinegar, toss, divide between plates and serve as a side dish.

Enjoy!

Nutrition: calories 90, fat 1, fiber 3, carbs 7, protein 2

## 261. Bell Peppers Mix

Preparation time: 10 minutes

Cooking time: 10 minutes

Servings: 2

Ingredients:

1 tablespoon olive oil

2 teaspoons garlic powder

2 red bell peppers, chopped

2 yellow bell peppers, chopped

2 orange bell peppers, chopped

Black pepper to the taste

Directions:

Heat up a pan with the oil over medium-high heat, add all the bell peppers, stir and cook for 5 minutes.

Add garlic powder and black pepper, stir, cook for 5 minutes, divide between plates and serve as a side dish.

Enjoy!

Nutrition: calories 145, fat 3, fiber 5, carbs 5, protein 8

## 262. Sweet Potato Mash

Preparation time: 10 minutes

Cooking time: 1 hour

Servings: 6

Ingredients:

¼ cup olive oil

3 pounds sweet potatoes

Black pepper to the taste

Directions:

Arrange the sweet potatoes on a lined baking sheet, introduce in the oven, bake at 375 degrees F for 1 hour, cool them down, peel, mash them and put them in a bowl.

Add black pepper and the oil, whisk well, divide between plates and serve as a side dish.

Enjoy!

Nutrition: calories 140, fat 1, fiber 4, carbs 6, protein 4

## 263. Bok Choy Mix

Preparation time: 10 minutes

Cooking time: 15 minutes

Servings: 4

Ingredients:

2 tablespoons olive oil

3 tablespoons coconut aminos

1-inch ginger, grated

A pinch of red pepper flakes

4 bok choy heads, cut into quarters

2 garlic cloves, minced

1 tablespoon sesame seeds, toasted

Directions:

Heat up a pan with the olive oil over medium heat, add coconut aminos, garlic, pepper flakes and ginger, stir and cook for 3-4 minutes.

Add the bok choy and the sesame seeds, toss, cook for 5 minutes more, divide between plates and serve as a side dish.

Enjoy!

Nutrition: calories 140, fat 2, fiber 2, carbs 4, protein 6

## 264. Flavored Turnips Mix

Preparation time: 10 minutes

Cooking time: 15 minutes

Servings: 4

Ingredients:

1 tablespoon lemon juice

Zest of 2 oranges, grated

16 ounces turnips, sliced

3 tablespoons olive oil

1 tablespoon rosemary, chopped

Black pepper to the taste

Directions:

Heat up a pan with the oil over medium-high heat, add turnips, stir and cook for 5 minutes.

Add lemon juice, black pepper, orange zest and rosemary, stir, cook for 10 minutes more, divide between plates and serve as a side dish.

Enjoy!

Nutrition: calories 130, fat 1, fiber 2, carbs 8, protein 4

## 265. Lemony Fennel Mix

Preparation time: 10 minutes

Cooking time: 0 minutes

Servings: 4

Ingredients:

3 tablespoons lemon juice

1 pound fennel, chopped

2 tablespoons olive oil

A pinch of black pepper

Directions:

In a salad bowl, mix fennel with and black pepper, oil and lemon juice, toss well, divide between plates and serve as a side dish.

Enjoy!

Nutrition: calories 130, fat 1, fiber 1, carbs 7, protein 7

## 266. Simple Cauliflower Mix

Preparation time: 10 minutes

Cooking time: 35 minutes

Servings: 4

Ingredients:

6 cups cauliflower florets

2 teaspoons sweet paprika

2 cups chicken stock

¼ cup avocado oil

Black pepper to the taste

Directions:

In a baking dish, combine the cauliflower with stock, oil, black pepper and paprika, toss, introduce in the oven and bake at 375 degrees F for 35 minutes.

Divide between plates and serve as a side dish.

Enjoy!

Nutrition: calories 180, fat 3, fiber 2, carbs 46, protein 6

## 267. Coconut Butternut Squash Mix

Preparation time: 10 minutes

Cooking time: 40 minutes

Servings: 4

Ingredients:

2 tablespoons coconut oil, melted

2 pounds butternut squash, peeled, seeded and cubed

2 teaspoons cilantro, chopped

A pinch of black pepper

Directions

In a bowl, mix squash with oil, cilantro and pepper, toss to coat well, spread on a lined baking sheet, bake in the oven at 425 degrees F for 40 minutes, divide between plates and serve as a side dish.


Enjoy!

Nutrition: calories 170, fat 1, fiber 2, carbs 6, protein 6

## 268. Cinnamon Butternut Squash Mix

Preparation time: 10 minutes

Cooking time: 30 minutes

Servings: 4

Ingredients:

½ teaspoon cinnamon powder

2 tablespoons olive oil

2 apples, peeled, cored and cubed

1 and ½ pounds butternut squash, peeled, seeded and cubed

Directions:

In a baking dish, mix apples with squash, cinnamon and oil, toss to coat, bake in the oven at 350 degrees F for 30 minutes, divide between plates and serve as a side dish.

Enjoy!

Nutrition: calories 150, fat 2, fiber 2, carbs 8, protein 7

## 269. Walnuts Zucchini Spaghetti

Preparation time: 10 minutes

Cooking time: 10 minutes

Servings: 4

Ingredients:

1/3 cup olive oil

4 zucchinis, cut with a spiralizer

¼ cup basil, chopped

Black pepper to the taste

½ cup walnuts, chopped

2 garlic cloves, minced

Directions:

Heat up a pan with the oil over medium-high heat, add zucchini spaghetti and garlic, stir and cook for 5 minutes.

Add basil, walnuts and black pepper, stir, cook for 5 minutes more, divide between plates and serve as a side dish.

Enjoy!

Nutrition: calories 150, fat 2, fiber 4, carbs 7, protein 10

## 270. Bacon Cabbage Mix

Preparation time: 10 minutes

Cooking time: 20 minutes

Servings: 4

Ingredients:

1 green cabbage head, shredded

2 tablespoons water

6 ounces bacon, chopped

A pinch of black pepper

1 teaspoon sweet paprika

1 tablespoon dill, chopped

Directions:

Heat up a pan over medium-high heat, add bacon and cook for 10 minutes.

Add the cabbage, the water, black pepper, paprika and dill, toss, cook for 10 minutes, divide between plates and serve as a side dish.

Enjoy!

Nutrition: calories 140, fat 2, fiber 6, carbs 8, protein 6

## 271. Celery And Kale Mix

Preparation time: 10 minutes

Cooking time: 20 minutes

Servings: 4

Ingredients:

2 celery stalks, chopped

5 cups kale, torn

3 tablespoons water

1 tablespoon olive oil

Directions:

Heat up a pan with the oil over medium-high heat, add celery, stir and cook for 10 minutes.

Add kale and water, toss, cook for 10 minutes more, divide between plates and serve as a side dish.

Enjoy!

Nutrition: calories 140, fat 1, fiber 2, carbs 6, protein 6

## 272. Kale And Red Chard Mix

Preparation time: 10 minutes

Cooking time: 10 minutes

Servings: 4

Ingredients:

5 cups kale, roughly chopped

1 and ½ tablespoons olive oil

3 cups red chard, chopped

2 tablespoons water

Black pepper to the taste

Directions:

Heat up a pan with the oil over medium-high heat, add red chard, kale and water, stir and cook for 10 minutes.

Add black pepper to the taste, toss, divide between plates and serve as a side dish.

Enjoy!

Nutrition: calories 150, fat 1, fiber 5, carbs 10, protein 7

## 273. Coconut Chard

Preparation time: 10 minutes

Cooking time: 10 minutes

Servings: 2

Ingredients:

Juice of ½ lemon

1 tablespoon olive oil

12 ounces canned coconut milk

1 bunch chard

Black pepper to the taste

Directions:

Heat up a pan with the oil over medium-high heat, add chard, stir and cook for 5 minutes.

Add lemon juice, black pepper and coconut milk, stir, cook for 5 minutes more, divide between plates and serve as a side dish.

Enjoy!

Nutrition: calories 150, fat 3, fiber 4, carbs 6, protein 7

## 274. Cauliflower And Eggplant Mix

Preparation time: 10 minutes

Cooking time: 40 minutes

Servings: 4

Ingredients:

1 cauliflower head, florets separated

1 small eggplant, cubed

1 small red bell pepper, cubed

5 tablespoons olive oil

4 tablespoons lemon juice

1 teaspoon garlic powder

Black pepper to the taste

½ teaspoon cumin powder

Directions:

Arrange eggplant, cauliflower and bell pepper pieces on a lined baking sheet, drizzle the oil, add lemon juice, garlic powder, black pepper and cumin, toss, introduce in the oven, bake at 400 degrees F for 40 minutes, divide between plates and serve as a side dish.

Enjoy!

Nutrition: calories 130, fat 1, fiber 3, carbs 7, protein 7

## 275. Artichoke Side Salad

Preparation time: 10 minutes

Cooing time: 0 minutes

Servings: 4

Ingredients:

4 ounces prosciutto, cut into strips

1 big romaine lettuce head, torn

½ cup artichoke hearts, roughly chopped

½ cup pickled hot peppers, chopped

½ cup black olives, pitted and chopped

For the dressing:

1 tablespoon parsley, chopped

1 garlic clove, minced

1 teaspoon oregano, dried

Black pepper to the taste

¾ cup olive oil

¼ cup red wine vinegar

Directions:

In a bowl, mix parsley with garlic, oregano, black pepper, oil and vinegar and whisk well.

In a salad bowl, mix prosciutto with romaine lettuce, artichoke hearts, hot peppers and olives, add the salad dressing, toss, divide between plates and serve as a side dish..

Enjoy!

Nutrition: calories 130, fat 1, fiber 2, carbs 7, protein 4

# Chapter 7. Dessert

## 276. Warm Berry Compote

 Preparation Time: 35 Minutes

Servings: 5

Ingredients:

2 cups blueberries

1 cup blackberries

2 cups strawberries

1 cup granulated sugar

1 tsp vanilla extract

½ cup coconut oil, softened

Directions:

Plug in your instant pot and press the 'Sauté' button. Add sugar and ½ cup of water. Simmer for 10-12 minutes or until sugar dissolves.

Now add the remaining ingredients and pour in 3 cups of water. Seal the lid and press the 'Manual' button. Set the timer for 25 minutes.

When done, release the pressure naturally and open the lid. Optionally add 1 tablespoon of freshly squeezed lemon juice.

Refrigerate for one hour before serving.

## 277. Warm Apple Dessert

Preparation Time: 15 Minutes

Servings: 3

Ingredients:

1 lb apples, peeled and chopped into bite-sized pieces

¼ cup quick oats

¼ cup almond butter

¼ cup coconut flour

1 tsp ground cinnamon

¼ tsp ground nutmeg

2 tbsp agave nectar

Directions:

Rinse and peel the apples. Chop into bite-sized pieces and place in your instant pot. Add one cup of water, cinnamon and nutmeg. Set aside.

Meanwhile, melt the butter in a small saucepan and add oats, coconut flour, and sugar. Stir well and simmer for 5 minutes.

Transfer the mixture to your instant pot and add agave nectar. Seal the lid and press the 'Manual' button. Cook for 8 minutes.

When done, release the pressure naturally and open the lid. Let it sit for 5 minutes before serving.

## 278. French Pear Pie

 Preparation Time: 45 Minutes

Servings: 5

Ingredients:

1 lb pears, peeled and sliced

2 tbsp freshly squeezed lemon juice

1 ½ cup brown sugar

½ tsp ground nutmeg

¾ cup coconut oil

1 cup all-purpose flour

7-inch egg-free pie crust

Directions:

Place pears in a large bowl and sprinkle with lemon juice and nutmeg. Stir well and set aside.

In another bowl, combine together flour, coconut oil, and one cup of sugar.

Line a 7-inches cake pan with parchment paper and place the crust in it. Sprinkle with the remaining sugar and top with pears. Finally, sprinkle with the sugar mixture.

Pour in two cups of water in your instant pot and set the steamer rack. Gently place the cake pan and close the lid.

Set the 'Manual' mode for 25 minutes.

When you hear the cooker's end signal, release the pressure naturally and open the lid.

Remove the pan and cool to a room temperature. Transfer to the fridge and cool completely before serving.

## 279. Apple and Cream Pie

Preparation Time: 50 Minutes

Servings: 8

Ingredients:

2 lbs apples, chopped

1 tsp ground cinnamon

¼ tsp ground nutmeg

1 tbsp lemon zest

¼ cup freshly squeezed lemon juice

½ cup silken tofu

¼ cup coconut cream

7-inches vegan pastry crust

Directions:

Roll out the pastry crust to approximately 7-inches circle and tightly wrap with plastic foil. Refrigerate for one hour.

Line a 7-inches round cake pan with some parchment paper and set aside.

In a large bowl, combine apples, cinnamon, nutmeg, lemon zest, and lemon juice. Stir well and set aside.

Place coconut cream and silken tofu in a large mixing bowl. With a paddle attachment on, mix well on high speed.

Finally, combine the pie mixture with the cream mixture and pour over the crust. Tightly wrap the entire pan with aluminum foil.

Plug in your instant pot and pour in 3 cups of water. Set the trivet and gently put the pie on top.

Close the cooker's lid and press the 'Manual' button. Set the timer for 40 minutes.

When done, release the pressure naturally and open the lid. Cool completely before serving.

## 280. Tarte Tatin

 Preparation Time: 60 Minutes

Servings: 5

Ingredients:

1 unbaked vegan pie crust, 7-inches

¾ cup brown sugar

¼ cup maple syrup

¼ cup almond butter

1 tbsp all-purpose flour

4 medium-sized Granny apples, chopped

Directions:

Plug in your instant pot and set the stainless steel insert. Add apples, butter, sugar, and maple syrup.

Press the 'Sauté' button and cook for 12-15 minutes, stirring constantly.

Remove the apples from your instant pot and set aside.

Grease a 7-inches round pan with some oil or butter and set aside.

Roll out the pie crust on a lightly floured work surface. Gently transfer to the prepared pan and top with the apple mixture. Optionally drizzle with some freshly squeezed lemon juice and tightly wrap with aluminum foil.

Pour 2 cups of water in your instant pot and set the steam rack. Place the pan on top and seal the lid.

Press the 'Manual' mode and set the timer to 30 minutes.

When done, release the pressure naturally and open the lid.

Cool completely before serving.

## 281. Cinnamon Pancakes

 Preparation Time: 15 Minutes

Servings: 4

Ingredients:

1 cup all-purpose flour

1 tbsp egg replacement

1 cup coconut milk

1 tsp baking powder

1 tsp baking soda

1 tsp vanilla extract

1 tsp cinnamon, ground

½ tsp salt

2 tbsp vegetable oil

Directions:

In a large mixing bowl, combine flour, egg replacement, milk, baking powder, baking soda, vanilla extract, cinnamon, and salt. With a whisking attachment on, beat well on high speed until fully incorporated.

Plug in your instant pot and grease the stainless steel insert with some oil. Pres the 'Sauté' button.

Pour in ½ cup of the batter and cook until golden. Gently flip and continue to cook for 3-4 minutes.

Using a kitchen spatula, gently remove the pancake from your pot. Repeat the process with the remaining batter.

## 282. Chocolate Mousse

Preparation Time: 35 Minutes

Servings: 2

Ingredients:

2 cups coconut milk

½ cup maple syrup

1 tsp rum extract

½ cup semisweet vegan chocolate

¼ cup chopped almonds, for topping

Directions:

Plug in your instant pot and press the 'Sauté' button. Add coconut milk, maple syrup, and rum extract. Gently simmer for 10 minutes, stirring constantly. Now, add chocolate and continue to cook until the chocolate melts.

Press the 'Cancel' button and transfer the mixture in a large bowl. Cool to a room temperature.

Refrigerate until the mixture thickens. Optionally, top with chopped almonds.

## 283. Blueberry Clafoutis

Preparation Time: 35 Minutes

Servings: 6

Ingredients:

1 lb fresh blueberries

3 tbsp egg replacement

1 cup brown sugar

1 ¼ cup coconut milk

1 tsp vanilla extract

¾ cup all-purpose flour

¼ cup coconut flour

1 tsp salt

Directions:

Grease a round 7-inches cake pan with some oil and line with parchment paper.

Spread the blueberries over the pan and sprinkle with coconut flour. Set aside.

Whisk together coconut milk, sugar, egg replacement, and vanilla extract. Transfer to a mixing bowl and beat well on high speed. Slowly pour in the flour and continue to beat for 2 minutes.

Pour the mixture over the blueberries and flatten the surface using a kitchen spatula. Cover with aluminum foil.

Plug in your instant pot and pour in 2 cups of water. Set the steam rack and place the pan on top. Seal the lid and press the 'Manual' mode. Set the timer to 25 minutes.

When done, release the pressure naturally and open the lid. Gently remove the pan and cool to a room temperature.

Refrigerate for one hour.

## 284. Banana Bread

 Preparation Time: 35 Minutes

Servings: 6

Ingredients:

3 large bananas

¾ cup almond butter

1 cup brown sugar

2 tbsp chia seeds

½ tsp salt

2 cups all-purpose flour

1 ½ tsp baking soda

Directions:

Grease a round baking pan with some oil and line with parchment paper. Grease a round 7-inches cake pan with some oil and line with parchment paper.

Spread the blueberries over the pan and sprinkle with coconut flour. Set aside.

Whisk together coconut milk, sugar, egg replacement, and vanilla extract. Transfer to a mixing bowl and beat well on high speed. Slowly pour in the flour and continue to beat for 2 minutes.

Pour the mixture over the blueberries and flatten the surface using a kitchen spatula. Cover with aluminum foil.

Plug in your instant pot and pour in 2 cups of water. Set the steam rack and place the pan on top. Seal the lid and press the 'Manual' mode. Set the timer to 25 minutes.

When done, release the pressure naturally and open the lid. Gently remove the pan and cool to a room temperature.

Refrigerate for one hour.

## 285. Pumpkin Bars

Preparation Time: 40 Minutes

Servings: 8

Ingredients:

7 oz pumpkin, cut into cubes

1 medium-sized banana

1 tbsp flaxseed

½ tsp cinnamon, ground

1 tbsp dried cranberries

½ cup almond meal

1 tbsp lemon zest

Directions:

Place pumpkin in your instant pot and pour in enough water to cover. Seal the lid and set the steam release handle. Press the 'Stew' button. When you hear the cooker's end signal, perform a quick release and open the lid. It should be fork tender but not overcooked.

Line some parchment paper over a round baking pan and set aside.

In a large mixing bowl, combine the ingredients and mix well with your hands. Spread the mixture over a baking dish and press with your hands to flatten the surface as much as possible.

Pour 2 cups of water in your instant pot and set the steam rack. Place the pan on top and seal the lid.

Set the steam release handle and press the 'Manual' button. Set the timer to 15 minutes.

When done, perform a quick release and open the lid. Remove the pan and cool to a room temperature.

Using a sharp knife, cut into desired size.

Refrigerate for 2 hours before serving.

## 286. Cider Cake

Preparation Time: 50 Minutes

Servings: 6

Ingredients:

3 cups all-purpose flour

2 tsp baking powder

1 tsp baking soda

1 tsp cinnamon

1 tsp salt

1 ½ cup sugar

2 tbsp coconut oil, melted

¾ cup pumpkin puree

1 cup apple cider

¾ cup oil

1 tsp rum extract

3 tbsp egg substitute

Directions:

Grease a round cake pan with coconut oil and sprinkle with some flour. Set aside.

In a large mixing bowl, combine flour, baking powder, baking soda, cinnamon, and salt. Mix well and add sugar, oil, apple cider, pumpkin puree, egg substitute, and rum extract. With a paddle attachment on, beat well on high speed – for 3 minutes.

Transfer the batter in the prepared pan and wrap with aluminum foil.

Plug in your instant pot and pour in 2 cups of water. Set the trivet and place the pan on top.

Seal the lid and set the steam release handle. Press the 'Manual' button and set the timer for 40 minutes.

When done, release the pressure naturally and open the lid.

Remove the pan and cool to a room temperature. Slice the cake into 8 pieces and refrigerate.

# 287. Blueberry Muffins

Preparation Time: 20 Minutes

Servings: 6

Ingredients:

½ cup all-purpose flour

1 tsp baking powder

¼ tsp salt

¼ cup brown sugar

3 tbsp almond butter

1 large banana

5 tbsp blueberries

½ cup coconut milk

Directions:

Place all dry ingredients in a large mixing bowl. Whisk together and add almond butter, coconut milk, and chopped banana. With a paddle attachment on, beat well on high speed.

Finally, add blueberries and mix again.

Grease a 6-cup silicon muffin pan with some oil and divide the batter between cups.

Plug in your instant pot and pour in 1 cup of water. Place the trivet inside and add muffins.

Seal the lid and set the steam release handle. Press the 'Manual' button and set the timer for 15 minutes.

When done, perform a quick release and open the lid.

Cool muffins completely before serving.

## 288. Lemon Glazed Cake

Preparation Time: 60 Minutes

Servings: 8

Ingredients:

1 ½ cup all-purpose flour

½ tsp baking powder

1/8 tsp baking soda

¼ tsp salt

1 1/3 cup brown sugar

1 tbsp lemon zest

¾ cup almond butter

2 cups silken tofu

1 ½ tsp vanilla extract

3 tbsp egg replacement

2 cups powdered sugar

¼ cup lemon juice

Directions:

In a large mixing bowl, combine flour, baking powder, baking soda, salt, brown sugar, and lemon zest. Mix well and add almond butter. With a paddle attachment, beat well on high speed. Now add the silken tofu, vanilla extract, and egg replacement.

Continue to beat on high speed – for 3 minutes.

Grease a round cake pan with oil and pour the batter in it.

Plug in your instant pot and pour in 2 cups of water. Set the steam rack and place the pan on top.

Seal the lid and set the steam release handle. Press the 'Manual' button and set the timer for 25 minutes.

When done, release the pressure naturally and open the lid.

Meanwhile, beat together powdered sugar and lemon juice. Refrigerate for 30 minutes.

Remove the cake from the pan and cool to a room temperature. Using a kitchen spatula, spread the lemon glaze mixture over your cake and refrigerate for 2 hours.

## 289. Coconut Orange Brownies

Preparation Time: 60 Minutes

Servings: 6

Ingredients:

¾ cup brown sugar

¼ cup raisins

2 tbsp breadcrumbs

¾ cup walnuts, minced

¼ cup orange zest

4 tbsp egg replacement

1 cup natural cane sugar

1 cup water

1 tsp rum extract

2 cups coconut cream

Directions:

In a large mixing bowl, combine sugar, raisins, breadcrumbs, walnuts, orange zest, and egg replacement. Beat well on high speed until fully incorporated. Refrigerate the mixture for 30 minutes.

Meanwhile, plug in your instant pot and press the 'Sauté' button. Add cane sugar, water, and rum. Cook for 7-10 minutes, or until sugar dissolves.

Press the 'Cancel' button and remove the mixture. Let it stand in the fridge.

Now line a 7-inches round pan with some parchment paper and sprinkle with some flour. Remove the batter from the fridge and wrap with aluminum foil.

Pour 2 cups of water in your instant pot and place the steam rack. Put the pan on top and seal the lid. Press the 'Manual' mode and set the timer to 15 minutes.

When done, release the pressure naturally and open the lid. Remove the cake and drizzle with the cane mixture.

Top with coconut cream and chill for one hour before serving.

## 290. Pumpkin Squares

 Preparation Time: 50 Minutes

Servings: 8

Ingredients:

2 cups all-purpose flour

2 tsp baking powder

1 tsp cinnamon, ground

¼ cup almonds, minced

3 tbsp egg replacement

2/3 cup coconut oil, melted

¾ cup sugar

1 tsp vanilla extract

2 cups pumpkin puree

1 tbsp orange zest

2/3 cup silken tofu

1 tbsp chia seeds

1 tsp rum extract

½ cup brown sugar

Directions:

In a medium-sized bowl, combine silken tofu, chia seeds, rum extract, brown sugar and three tablespoons of water. Using a hand mixer, beat well until light and creamy. Refrigerate for 30 minutes.

In another bowl, combine flour, baking powder, cinnamon, almonds, egg replacement, coconut oil, sugar, vanilla extract, pumpkin puree, and orange zest. Beat well with a hand mixer on medium speed.

Line a square cake pan with some parchment paper and pour the batter in it. Flatten the surface with a kitchen spatula and wrap with aluminum foil.

Plug in your instant pot and pour in 2 cups of water. Set the trivet and place the pan on top. Seal the lid and set the steam release handle. Press the 'Manual' mode for 30 minutes.

When done, release the pressure naturally and remove the pan from the pot. Chill to a room temperature and top with chilled tofu mixture.

Refrigerate overnight.

## 291. Easy Plum Pudding

 Preparation Time: 35 Minutes

Servings: 8

Ingredients:

3 lbs plums, pits removed

2 cups brown sugar

1 tsp vanilla extract

¼ cup freshly squeezed orange juice

Directions:

Place the plums in a large colander. Rinse them thoroughly under cold running water and drain. Remove the pits and place in your instant pot.

Add the remaining ingredients and pour in 2 cups of water.

Seal the lid and set the steam release handle. Press the 'Manual' button and set the timer for 20 minutes.

When you hear the cooker's end signal, perform a quick release and open the lid. Pour the mixture in 8 serving bowls and refrigerate for one hour.

## 292. Coconut Cake

Preparation Time: 35 Minutes

Servings: 8

Ingredients:

2 cups coconut cream

1 ½ cup brown sugar

1 ½ cup almond flour

1 cup coconut oil, melted

1 cup coconut flour

1 tsp baking soda

1 cup dark vegan chocolate, chopped into chunks

Directions:

Combine coconut cream, brown sugar, almond flour, and baking soda in a large bowl. Stir with a wooden spatula until well combined. Gradually, add coconut oil and coconut flour. Mix well with a hand mixer on medium speed.

Line a 7-inches round baking pan with some parchment paper. Pour the batter in the prepared baking pan and wrap with aluminum foil.

Plug in your instant pot and add one cup of water. Set the trivet and put the pan on top.

Seal the lid and press the 'Manual' mode. Set the timer for 20 minutes.

Meanwhile, place chocolate chunks in a microwave safe bowl. Melt the chocolate.

When you hear the cooker's end signal, perform a quick release and remove the pan.

Drizzle the cake with chocolate and cool to a room temperature. Transfer to the fridge and cool completely.

## 293. Easy Fig Compote

 Preparation Time: 35 Minutes

Servings: 8

Ingredients:

1 lb fresh figs

10 oz fresh strawberries

2 large pears, chopped

3.5 oz raisins

3 tbsp of cornstarch

1 tsp cinnamon, ground

1 tsp cloves

174 cup sugar

1 lemon, juiced

Directions:

Wash and prepare the fruits for the compote.

Plug in your instant pot and simply combine all ingredients in the stainless steel insert. Pour about 3-4 cups of water : depending on how much liquid you wishand close the lid. Set the release steam handle and press "Manual" button. Set the timer to 30 minutes and cook on high pressure.

When done, press "Cancel" button and turn off the pot. Release the steam naturally. Let it stand for 10 minutes to chill before opening.

Enjoy!

## 294. Cranberry Lemon Blondie's

Preparation Time: 35 Minutes

Servings: 10

Ingredients:

2 cups whole wheat pastry flour

1 teaspoon dried thyme

3/4 cup sugar

3/4 cup nondairy milk

Zest of 1 lemon

Juice of 2 lemons

1/4 cup dried cranberries

1/2 teaspoon baking soda

1 teaspoon baking powder

1/2 teaspoon salt

1/2 teaspoon almond extract

1 teaspoon orange extract

3 tablespoons olive oil

Directions:

Mix together all the dry ingredients.

In a separate bowl, stir together the wet ingredients. Then, add the dry ingredients a little at a time until well combined.

Place a cup of water in the bottom of the instant pot, and then place a rack on top.

Spray a baking dish or loaf pan small enough to fit in your instant pot with nonstick spray.

Pour the brownie batter into the greased pan and lightly cover it with foil before lowering it onto the rack.

Seal the lid and cook on high for 20 minutes, quick releasing the pressure when it is finished.

## 295. Warm Winter Compote

 Preparation Time: 35 Minutes

Servings: 8

Ingredients:

1 lb fresh figs

7 oz Turkish figs

7 oz fresh cherries

7 oz plums

3.5 oz raisins

3 large apples

3 tbsp of cornstarch

1 tsp cinnamon, ground

1 tsp cloves

1 tsp powdered Stevia

1 lemon, juiced

3 cups of water

Directions:

Wash and prepare the fruits for the compote.

Plug in your instant pot and simply combine all ingredients in the stainless steel insert. Pour about 3-4 cups of water : depending on how much liquid you wishand close the lid. Set the release steam handle and press "Manual" button. Set the timer to 30 minutes and cook on high pressure.

When done, press "Cancel" button and turn off the pot. Release the steam naturally. Let it stand for 10 minutes to chill before opening.

Enjoy!

# 296. Sweet Heat Protein Brownies

Preparation Time:  Minutes

Servings: 12

Ingredients:

1 can black beans, drained and rinsed

2 bananas

3 tablespoons applesauce

1/2 cup instant oatmeal

1/2 cup chopped walnuts

1/4 cup agave nectar

1/2 cup cocoa powder

1/8 teaspoon cayenne pepper

1/2 teaspoon cinnamon

1/4 teaspoon chipotle chili powder

1 teaspoon vanilla extract

Directions:

Pulse the oatmeal in the food processor until it reaches a flour type consistency. Set aside in a large bowl.

Puree the rest of the ingredients in the food processor, and then combine the mixture with the oats and walnuts.

Place a cup of water in the bottom of the instant pot, and then place a rack on top.

Spray a baking dish or loaf pan small enough to fit in your instant pot with nonstick spray.

Pour the brownie batter into the greased pan and lightly cover it with foil before lowering it onto the rack.

Seal the lid and cook on high for 20 minutes, quick releasing the pressure when it is finished.

## 297. Pumpkin Spiced Pudding

Preparation Time: 15 Minutes

Servings: 6

Ingredients:

9 1/2 ounces firm tofu

2 1/2 cups pumpkin purée

1/2 cup maple syrup

2 tablespoons packed brown sugar

1 teaspoon cinnamon

1/2 teaspoon allspice

1/8 teaspoon ground ginger

1/8 teaspoon ground cloves

1/8 teaspoon nutmeg

Granola, for serving

Directions:

Puree all the ingredients in a food processor.

Pour into an oiled instant pot. Seal the lid and cook on low 5 minutes, then let the pressure release naturally.

Serve chilled and topped with granola and extra cinnamon.

## 298. Orange Tapioca Pudding

Preparation Time: 22 Minutes

Servings: 2

Ingredients:

1/3 cup tapioca pearls

1 3/4 cups nondairy milk

1/4 cup sugar

1 teaspoon orange extract

Zest from one orange

Pinch of salt

Directions:

Rinse the tapioca pearls, and then pour them into a baking dish that will fit in your pressure cooker. Stir in the rest of the ingredients.

Place a rack in the bottom of the instant pot, then place the instant pot safe baking dish on top of the rack.

Seal the lid and cook on high 8 minutes, then let the pressure release naturally.

For extra flavor, stir in your favorite fruit.

## 299. Pina Colada Rice Pudding

Preparation Time: 15 Minutes

Servings: 8

Ingredients:

2 cups fresh pineapple, chopped

1 1/2 cups Arborio rice

1 teaspoon vanilla extract

1 cups nondairy milk

10 ounces light coconut milk

1/2 cup agave nectar

Directions:

Spray the instant pot with nonstick spray.

Combine all the ingredients in the instant pot. Seal the lid and cook on high 5 minutes, then let the pressure release naturally.

## 300. Floral Tapioca Pudding

Preparation Time: 22 Minutes

Servings: 6

Ingredients:

3 1/2 cups plain or unsweetened nondairy milk

1/2 cup tapioca pearls

1/2 cup sugar

Pinch of salt

1 teaspoon vanilla extract

1 teaspoon food grade rosewater

Directions:

Rinse the tapioca pearls, then pour them into a baking dish that will fit in your pressure cooker. Stir in the rest of the ingredients.

Place a rack in the bottom of the instant pot, then place the instant pot safe baking dish on top of the rack.

Seal the lid and cook on high 8 minutes, then let the pressure release naturally.

## 301. Sweet Tea Cinnamon Poached Pears

Preparation Time: 20 Minutes

Servings: 4

Ingredients:

1 cup prepared black tea

4 pears, peeled and halved

1/2 cup brown sugar

1 teaspoon vanilla extract

1/8 teaspoon cinnamon

1/8 teaspoon salt

Directions:

Stir together the tea, brown sugar, vanilla, salt, and cinnamon.

Spray the instant pot with nonstick spray, then lay the pear halves in the bottom.

Pour the sauce on top. Seal the lid and cook on high 10 minutes, then let the pressure release naturally.

Serve garnished with additional brown sugar.

# 302. Citrus Apples with Rum and Tequila

Preparation Time: 30 Minutes

Servings: 4

Ingredients:

3 tablespoons rum

1 tablespoon tequila

4 apples, peeled and sliced

1 tablespoon brown sugar

Juice 3 tangerines

Zest of 2 tangerines

Juice of 1/2 lime

1/2 teaspoon ground ginger

1/4 teaspoon nutmeg

Directions:

Spray the instant pot with nonstick spray and lay the apple slices in the bottom.

Combine the rest of the ingredients in a separate bowl, then pour over the apples.

Seal the lid and cook on high 8 minutes, then let the pressure release naturally.

Remove the lid and switch to the sauté setting. Simmer for an additional 10 minutes to reduce the alcohol.

## 303. Appleberry Cobbler

Preparation Time: 50 Minutes

Servings: 4

Ingredients:

1/2-pint strawberries, washed and chopped

1/2-pint raspberries, washed

2 apples, peeled and chopped

2 pears, peeled and chopped

1 tablespoon lemon juice

1 teaspoon lemon zest

1 1/2 teaspoons baking powder

1 1/2 cups flour

1/2 cup oat bran

1/2 cup plus 1/3 cup sugar

1 tablespoon cornstarch

Pinch of salt

1/2 cup nondairy milk

3 tablespoons olive oil

1 teaspoon vanilla extract

Directions:

For the biscuits, mix the bran, 1/3 cup sugar, baking powder, flour, and salt in a large mixing bowl. Add the nondairy milk, vanilla, and olive oil to the dry ingredients and stir well.

Roll the biscuits onto a floured surface until they are about ½ inch thick. Cut out small circles of dough using a cookie cutter or a drinking glass. Set aside.

Spray the instant pot with nonstick spray. Add the fruit, lemon juice and zest, ½ cup sugar, and salt to the instant pot. Seal the lid and cook on high 8 minutes, then quick release the pressure.

Add cornstarch if the sauce is too thick.

Lay the biscuits on top of the fruit and switch the instant pot to the sauté setting. Loosely cover the instant pot so that the condensation does not soak the biscuits. Cook for about 30 minutes until biscuits are done.

# Chapter 8. 21 day meal plan

| DAY | BREAKFAST | MAINS | SNACK/DESSERT |
|---|---|---|---|
| 1. | Blueberry Quinoa Muffins | Basil and Garlic Seitan Roast | Warm Apple Dessert |
| 2. | Mini Frittatas | Beet Greens with Tofu Chops | French Pear Pie |
| 3. | Chocolate Muffins | BBQ Baked Tempeh Chops | Apple and Cream Pie |
| 4. | Pumpkin Chocolate Chip Quinoa Muffins | Chipotle-Coffee Tempeh Chops | Cinnamon Pancakes |
| 5. | Baked Eggs with Creamy Collard Greens | Mushroom Crackling with Coconut Creamed Kale | Warm Berry Compote |
| 6. | Ananas Quinoa | Tofu with Morels | Citrus Apples with Rum and Tequila |
| 7. | Blueberries Coconut Milk Yogurt | Special Jambalaya | Sweet Tea Cinnamon Poached Pears |
| 8. | Breakfast Stuffed Sweet Potatoes | Simple Tofu Dish | Floral Tapioca Pudding |
| 9. | Pumpkin Coffeecake Oatmeal | Delicious Butternut Squash Soup | Pina Colada Rice Pudding |
| 10. | Cilantro Lime Quinoa | Amazing Mushroom Stew | Pumpkin Spiced Pudding |

|  | | | |
|---|---|---|---|
| 11. | Broccoli Frittata with Peppers | Indian Lentils | Orange Tapioca Pudding |
| 12. | Slow Cook Barley with Apples | Rich Beans Soup | Sweet Heat Protein Brownies |
| 13. | Cottage cheese Stuffed Avocado | Incredibly Tasty Pizza | Lemon Glazed Cake |
| 14. | Burritos | Amazing Potato Dish | Banana Bread |
| 15. | Carrot Cake Quinoa | Delicious Baked Beans | Chocolate Mousse |
| 16. | Creamy Masala Millet | Textured Sweet Potatoes and Lentils Delight | Tarte Tatin |
| 17. | Veggie Quiche | Classic Black Beans Chili | Cider Cake |
| 18. | Nutmeg Banana Quinoa | Mushroom Tofu Meatballs with Coconut Parsnip Mash | Pumpkin Bars |
| 19. | Breakfast Potatoes | Red Wine Braised Mushroom | Coconut Orange Brownies |
| 20. | Quinoa Burrito Bowls | Herbed Lemon Garlic Tempeh | Blueberry Clafoutis |
| 21. | Butternut Squash Breakfast Bowls | Herby Lemon Greek Tenderloin | Blueberry Muffins |

# Conclusion

Without following these recipes to the latter and making sure that we actually and eventually adopt them, then we are in for more dangerous journeys, especially when our diets are concerned. We will be digging our graves when we fail to embrace this plant-based diet meal plan. The later is caused by the fact that there have been several cases of people just dying of food-related diseases such as obesity, heart attacks, and even fatigue. An excellent way to stop all these is to migrate completely from our current diet and look for ways to embrace this plant-based diet. By doing this, then issues of deaths will be reduced. The effects of medication and other forms of illness will be a thing of the past.